Pharmaceutical Engineering Drawing

For B. Pharmacy Students

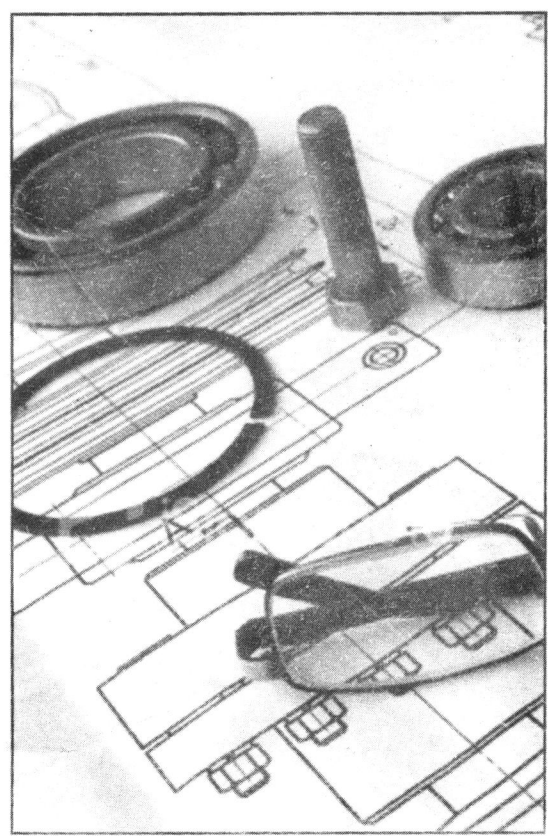

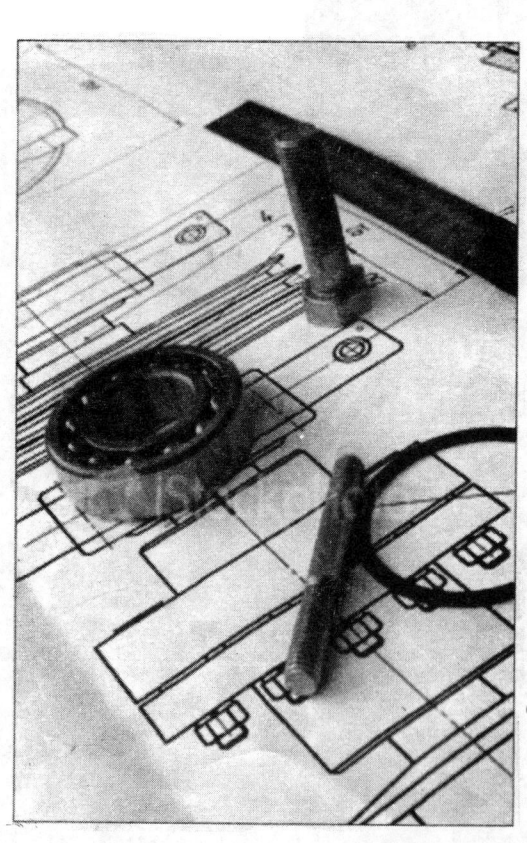

Pharmaceutical Engineering Drawing

For B. Pharmacy Students

Edited by:

Rajesh Kumar Nema
Director
SD College of Pharmacy and Vocational Studies
Muzaffarnagar, UP

Kamal Singh Rathore
Senior Lecturer
BN Girls College of Pharmacy
Udaipur, Rajasthan

C.S. Bhan
Principal
MGCPS, Jaipur, Rajasthan

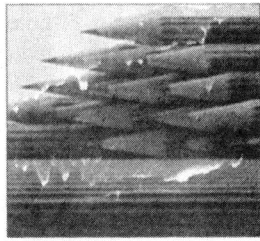

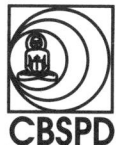

CBSPD

CBS Publishers & Distributors Pvt Ltd

New Delhi • Bengaluru • Chennai • Kochi • Kolkata • Lucknow • Mumbai
Hyderabad • Jharkhand • Nagpur • Patna • Pune • Uttarakhand

Pharmaceutical Engineering Drawing

ISBN: 978-81-239-1614-9

First Edition: 2008
Reprint: 2012, 2018, 2019, 2020, **2025**

Published by **Satish Kumar Jain** and produced by **Varun Jain** for

CBS Publishers & Distributors Pvt Ltd

4819/XI Prahlad Street, 24 Ansari Road, Daryaganj, New Delhi 110 002, India.
Ph: 011-23266838, 23289259   Website: www.cbspd.com
       e-mail: delhi@cbspd.com

Corporate Office: 204 FIE, Industrial Area, Patparganj, Delhi 110 092
Ph: 011-4934 4934   Fax: 011-4934 4935
       e-mail: publishing@cbspd.com; publicity@cbspd.com

Branches

- **Bengaluru:** Seema House 2975, 17th Cross, KR Road, Banasankari 2nd Stage, Bengaluru 560 070, Karnataka, India
  Ph: +91-80-26771678/79   Fax: +91-80-26771680   e-mail: bangalore@cbspd.com
- **Chennai:** 7, Subbaraya Street, Shenoy Nagar, Chennai 600 030, Tamil Nadu, India
  Ph: +91-44-26680620, 26681266   Fax: +91-44-42032115   e-mail: chennai@cbspd.com
- **Kochi:** 42/1325, 1326, Power House Road, Opp KSEB, Power House, Ernakulum Kochi 682 018, Kerala, India
  Ph: +91-484-4059061-65,67   Fax: +91-484-4059065   e-mail: kochi@cbspd.com
- **Kolkata:** 147, Hind Ceramics Compound, 1st Floor, Nilgunj Road, Belghoria, Kolkata-700056, West Bengal, India
  Ph: +033-25633055, 033-25633056   e-mail: kolkata@cbspd.com
- **Lucknow:** Basement, Khushnuma Complex, 7 Meerabai Marg (Behind Jawahar Bhawan), Lucknow-226001, UP, India
  Ph: +0522-4000032   e-mail: tiwari.lucknow@cbspd.com
- **Mumbai:** PWD Shed, Gala no 25/26, Ramchandra Bhatt Marg, Next to JJ Hospital Gate no. 2, Opp. Union Bank of India, Noorbaug, Mumbai-400009, Maharashtra, India
  Ph: 022-66661880/89   e-mail: mumbai@cbspd.com

Representatives

Hyderabad	0-9885175004	Jharkhand	0-9811541605	Nagpur	0-8692091830
Patna	0-9334159340	Pune	0-9664372571	Uttarakhand	0-9716462459

Printed at Neekunj Print Process, Haryana, India

Preface

We are very happy to introduce the book **Pharmaceutical Engineering Drawing** *for B. Pharm. Students*. The subject matter of this book covers the syllabi of pharmaceutical engineering drawing for B. Pharmacy course in various universities. This book covers lettering, lines and dimensioning, sheet layout, symbols of materials, free hand sketching, construction of scales, geometrical drawing, principles of projection, first angle and third angle methods of projection, isometric views, sectional views, nuts and bolts, valves, pipe joints, rivets and riveted joints, assembly drawings, and flow diagrams.

As this subject is not a part of the main stream of the course, we have, therefore, tried to explain the subject and techniques methodically and step-by-step in a way that is simple, and easy to understand and follow.

Suggestions and comments from the teachers and students to improve the value of this book are always welcome.

Rajesh Kumar Nema
Kamal Singh Rathore
CS Bhan

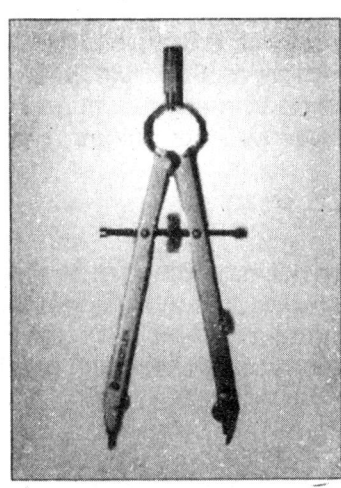

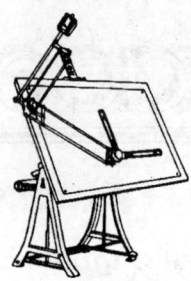

The Authors

Rajesh Kumar Nema

is currently Director, SD College of Pharmacy, Muzaffarnagar, UP. He is an eminent professor of pharmaceutical chemistry with more than 20 years of teaching experience, including 6 years of postgraduate experience. Prof Nema earned his B Pharm and M Pharm from Dr HS Gaur Vishwavidyalya, Sagar, and Ph D from Mohan Lal Sukhadia University, Udaipur. He has earlier worked as Acting Principal, BNPG College of Pharmacy, Udaipur, for two years. He was elected as President, Association of Pharmaceutical Teachers of India (Rajasthan State Branch). He has written several books and book chapters. He has attended various national and international conferences. He is a life member of IPA, ISTE, IHPA, APTI, IPGA.

Kamal Singh Rathore

is presently a senior lecturer at BN Girls College of Pharmacy, Udaipur. Having passed his M Pharm (pharmaceutics) from BN College of Pharmacy, MLS University, Udaipur, in 2005. Mr Rathore also holds an MBA degree from FMS, Udaipur, and served as a management trainer for 2 years in Zydus Cadila and Laderle. Mr Rothore has teaching experiences over 5 years and has written 20 research and review articles most of which have been published in international and national repute. He is a member of IPA, APTI, FIP, etc. He has presented international papers at Cairo and Kathmandu.

CS Bhan

is currently Principal at MGCPS, Jaipur. He has specialisation in pharmaceutical chemistry. He has a teaching experience of 17 years. Prof Bhan has held a number of administrative positions as HoD/ Principal in a number of pharmacy institutions in Rajasthan. He is life member of APTI, IHPA and has attended a number of conferences at national level. He is known for his teaching and administrative skills.

Contents

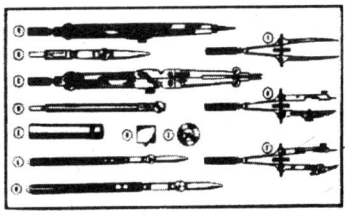

❑ **Geometry**: Drawing shows the shape of the object, represented as views, how the object will look when it is viewed from various standard directions such as from front, from top, from side, etc.

❑ **Dimensions**: The size of the object is captured in various units.

❑ **Tolerances**: The allowable variations for each dimension.

❑ **Material:** Represents the item is made-up of which material.

❑ **Finishing**: Specifies the surface quality of the item, e.g. a mass-marketed product usually requires a much higher surface quality than, say, a component that goes inside the industrial machinery.

❑ A variety of line styles graphically represents physical objects. Types of lines include the following:

- **Visible lines** are continuous lines used to depict edges directly visible from a particular angle.
- Hidden – are short-dashed lines that may be used to represent edges that are not directly visible.
- **Centre lines** are alternately long- and short-dashed lines that may be used to represent the axes of circular features.
- **Cutting planes** are thin, medium-dashed lines, or thick alternately long and double short-dashed that may be used to define sections for section views.
- **Section lines** are thin lines in a pattern (pattern determined by the material being **cut/sectioned**) used to indicate surfaces in section views resulting from **cutting**. Section lines are commonly referred to as **crosshatching**.
- Lines can also be classified by a letter classification in which each line is given a letter.
- **Type A** lines show the outline of the feature of an object. They are the thickest lines on a drawing and done with a pencil softer than HB.
- **Type B** lines are dimension lines and are used for dimensioning, projecting, extending, or leaders. A harder pencil should be used such as a 2H.
- **Type C** lines are used for breaks when the whole object is not shown. They are freehand drawn and only for short breaks (2H pencil).
- **Type D** lines are similar to Type C, except they are zigzagged and only for longer breaks (2H pencil).
- **Type E** lines indicate hidden outlines of internal features of an object. They are dotted lines (2H pencil).
- **Type F** lines are used for drawings in electro technology (2H pencil).
- **Type G** lines are used for centre lines. They are dotted lines, but a long line of 10–20 mm, then a gap, then a small line of 2 mm, (2H pencil).
- **Type H** lines are the same as Type G, except that every second long line is thicker. They indicate the cutting plane of an object (2H pencil).
- **Type K** lines indicate the alternate positions of an object and the line taken by that object. They are drawn with a long line of 10–20 mm, then a small gap, then a small line of 2 mm, then a gap and then another small line (2H pencil).

Introduction

INTRODUCTION

Pharmaceutical engineering drawing is a universal graphic language of engineers and pharmacists and is used to develop and record their ideas by means of drawing. It is technical in nature, used to fully and clearly define requirements for engineered items and is created with standardized conventions for layout nomenclature, interpretation, appearance and size. Drawing cannot be spoken or read aloud. For all types of technical and geometrical drawing it is necessary to use instruments of good quality and high grade to get the required degree of accuracy.

Special Features of Pharmaceutical Engineering Drawings

Drawings convey the following information.

- **Geometry:** Drawing shows the shape of the object, represented as views, how the object will look when it is viewed from various standard directions such as from front, from top, from side, etc.
- **Dimensions:** The size of the object is captured in various units.
- **Tolerances:** The allowable variations for each dimension.
- **Finishing** specifies the surface quality of the item, e.g. a mass-marked product usually requires a much higher surface quality than, say, a component that goes inside an industrial machinery.

A variety of the styles graphically represent physical objects. Types of lines include the following.

- **Visible lines** are continuous lines used to depict edges directly visible from a particular angle.
- **Hidden** lines are short-dashed lines that may be used to represent edges that are not directly visible.
- **Centre lines** are alternatively long- and short-dashed lines that may be used to represent the axes of circular features.
- **Cutting plane** are thin, medium-dashed lines, or thick alternately long and double short-dashed that may be used to define sections for section views.

- **Section lines** are thin lines in a pattern (pattern determined by the material being **cut/sectioned**) used to indicate surfaces in section views resulting from **cutting**. Section lines are commonly referred to as **crosshatching**.

Lines can also be classified by a letter classification in which each line is given a letter.

- **Type A** lines show the outline of the feature of an object. They are the thickest lines on a drawing and done with a pencil softer than HB.
- **Type B** lines are dimension lines which are used for dimensioning, projecting, extending, or leaders. A harder pencil should be used such as a 2H.
- **Type C** lines are used for breaks when the whole object is not shown. They are freehand drawn and used only for short breaks (2H pencil).
- **Type D** lines are similar to Type C, except they are zigzagged and only for longer breaks (2H pencil).
- **Type E** lines indicate hidden outlines of internal features of an object. They are dotted lines (2H pencil).
- **Type F** lines are used for drawings in electro technology (2H pencil).
- **Type G** lines are used for centre lines. They are dotted lines, but a long line of 10–20 mm, then a gap, then a small line of 2 mm (2H pencil).
- **Type H** lines are the same as Type G, except that every second long line is thicker. They indicate the cutting plane of an object (2H pencil).
- **Type K** lines indicate the alternate positions of an object and the line taken by that object. They are drawn with a long line of 10–20 mm, then a small gap, then a small line of 2 mm, then a gap and then another small line (2H pencil).

DRAWING INSTRUMENTS

The students should procure a good set of the following drawing instruments of as superior quality as possible.

1. Drawing board
2. T-square
3. Set-square (30°, 45° and 60°)
4. Compass with pencil legs
5. Hair spring divider
6. Set of scales
7. Protractor
8. Drawing pencils of different grades, e.g. 2H, H, HB
9. Drawing papers (ivory sheets)
10. Drawing pins/adhesive tape
11. Eraser (rubber)
12. Duster

13. Sand paper
14. Paper cutter
15. Drafter

HOW TO START

Place drawing board on the stand in such a way that working edge of the drawing board must be on left side, on which T-square is made to slide on it. Fix a drawing sheet (Size: Approx. 56 cm × 36 cm) on the board with the help of drawing pins or adhesive tape in a way that upper line of the sheet should be parallel to the T-square. Drafter can be fitted on the left side of the board, so it can easily be moved all over the sheet. Draw border lines at equal distances of about 20–25 mm from the top, bottom and right-hand edges of the sheet and about 40 mm from the left hand edge (required for binding/filing the drawing sheets) on the sheet by using HB pencil and a title block/two title blocks (13 cm × 7 cm) on each lower corners of the sheet. If only one drawing or figure is to be drawn on a sheet, it should be drawn in the centre of the working space, otherwise the space should be divided into suitable blocks and each figure should be drawn in the centre of the respective blocks.

Set-squares

Set-squares (45°, 45° and 90°) and (90°, 60° and 30°) are used to draw all straight, perpendicular and parallel lines by sliding them on each other (Fig. 1.1). Horizontal

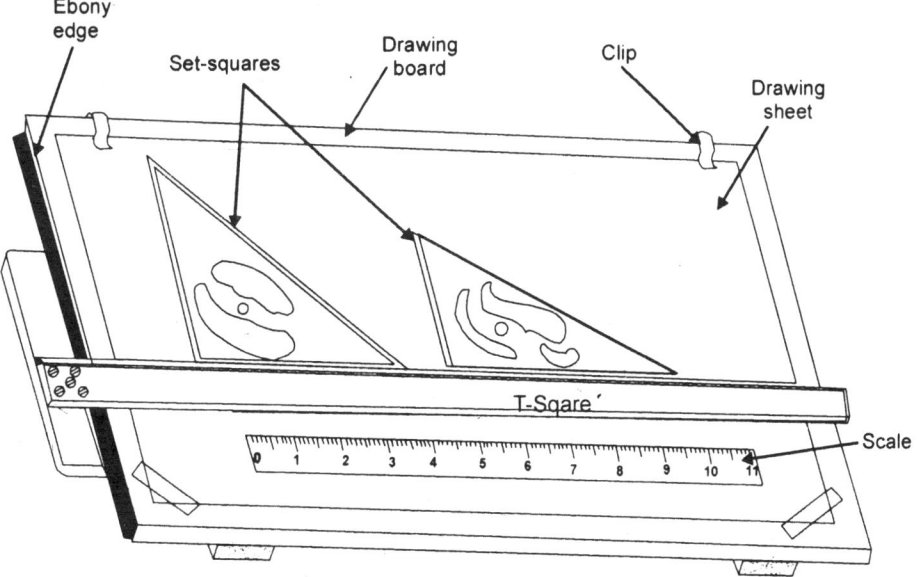

Fig. 1.1: *Drawing board, scale, T-square and set-squares*

lines are drawn by T-square while vertical lines with the help of set-square on the T-square (Fig.1.1). Angles of 15°, 30°, 45°, 60°, 75°, 90° and 105° are drawn with the help of set-squares. Angles of 15°, 75° and 105° can be drawn along with or simultaneously along with T-square.

Compass and Dividers

The compass is used for drawing circles and arcs of circles while dividers are used to divide curved or straight lines into desired number of equal part, to transfer dimensions from one part of the drawing to another part and to set-off given distances from the scale to the drawing (Fig.1.2).

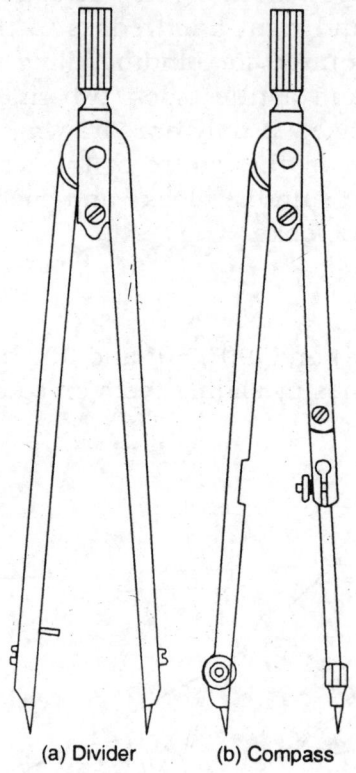

(a) Divider   (b) Compass

Fig. 1.2: Divider and compass

Scales

Scales are used for making measurements on the drawing paper accurately. Both the longer edges of the scales are marked with divisions of inches, centimeters, which are again subdivided into ten equal parts. A set of cardboard scales is available in a set of eight scales ($A - H$ and $M_1 - M_8$) which are used to transfer the true or relative dimensions of an object to the drawing.

Protractor

The protractor is used to draw or measure such angles which cannot be drawn with the help of set-squares (Fig.1.3). A circle can be divided into any number of equal parts with the help of protractor.

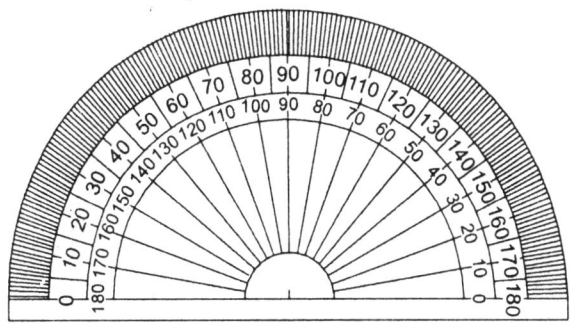

Fig. 1.3: *Protractor*

Drawing Papers

Nowadays drawing papers are available in many varieties. For ordinary pencil drawing the paper should be tough and strong, uniform in thickness and as white as possible. Paper of good quality and smooth surface is always advisable.

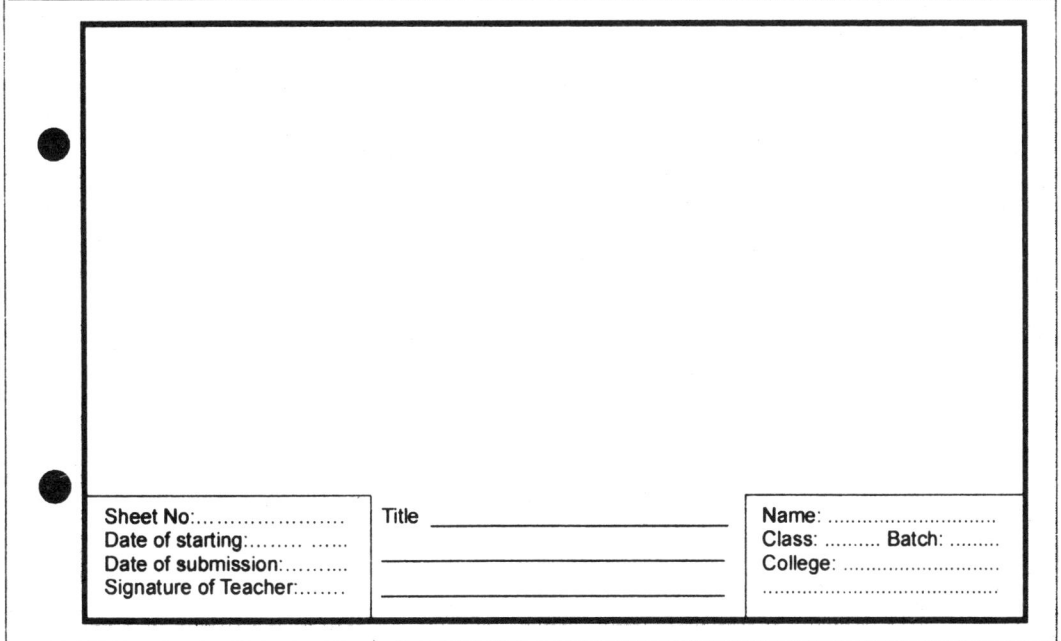

Fig. 1.4: *Layout of drawing sheet*

Drawing Pencils

Accuracy and appearance of a drawing mainly depend on the quality of the pencils used. The lines drawn should always be of uniform shade and thickness. The grade HB denotes the medium grade. When hardness of graphite increases, the shade becomes lighter (H, 2H, 3H, 4H, 5H, 6H, etc.) and when softness of graphite increases, the shade becomes darker (B, 2B, 3B, 4B, 5B, 6B, etc.). Generally, drawing should be made with hard grade pencils such as H or 2H pencil while soft grade pencils such as HB pencils are more suitable for lettering, dimensioning and for free-hand sketching. For uniform thickness of lines (*a*), the lead may be sharpened as conical point or chisel edge (*b*).

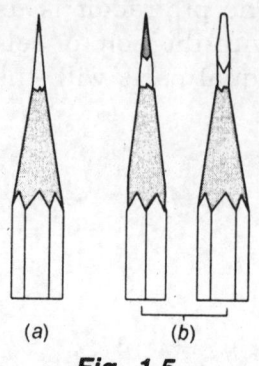

(a)   (b)

Fig. 1.5

The conical point is used for sketch work and for lettering while chisel edge is used for long, thin lines of uniform thickness.

Eraser (Rubber)

White soft rubber is most suitable kind of eraser for pencil drawings. Rubber should not spoil the surface of the drawing paper. Frequent use of rubber should be avoided.

Drawing Pins (Thumb Pins)

Thumb pins are used to fix the drawing paper on the drawing board by priming them on the board by thumbs. Sometimes clips or adhesive tapes are also used instead of pins.

Sand Paper

A piece of a fine sand paper is used for sharpening the point of the pencils either conical or chisel shape.

Duster

White towel cloth of convenient size or a napkin can be used as a duster. Before starting drawing, all instruments and materials should be thoroughly cleaned with the duster. After the use of rubber, the rubber crumbs formed should be swept away by the duster.

Drafter

Nowadays the uses and advantages of T-square, set-square, scales, and protractor are combined in the form of a drafter. One end of the drafter is clamped on the drawing board with the help of a screw at the left hand of the user (Fig. 1.6).

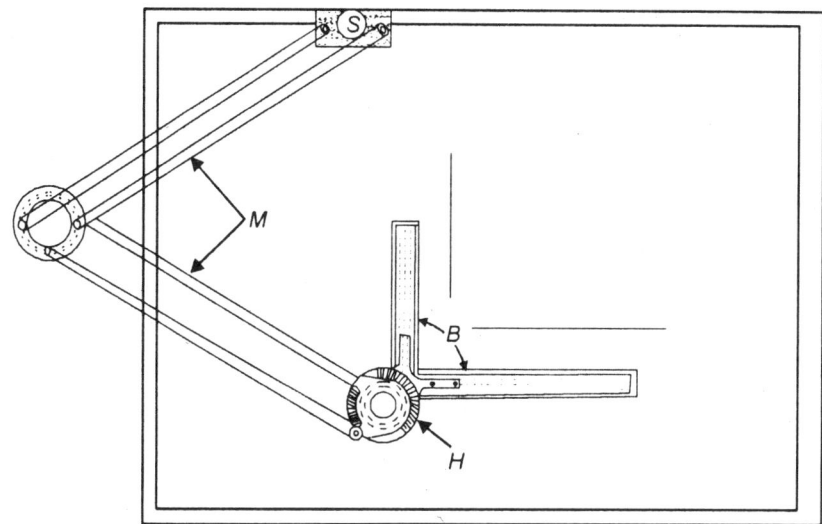

Fig. 1.6: *Drafter*

It has an adjustable head (*H*) having protractor marking and two blades set (*B*) having scales at right angles to each other and can be used as straight edge. The mechanism (*M*) keeps the two blades always parallel, wherever they may be moved on the board. First of all zero mark of the blades *B* is adjusted to the mark of the head (*H*) so that perpendicular or right angles can be drawn. Afterwards it can be rotated to any degree to get a desirable angle.

By means of the drafter, horizontal, vertical or inclined parallel lines of desired lengths can be drawn anywhere on the sheet at our convenience.

USEFUL TIPS TO BE WRITTEN ON THE DRAWING SHEET

1. The scale should never be used as a straight edge for drawing of lines.

2. Only upper edge of the T-square should be used for drawing of horizontal lines and should be used as a base for the set-square.

3. Any edge of the T-square should not be used for cutting the sheet with knife.

4. T-square should never be used as a hammer.

5. Drawing pencils should be well mended and points should be conical or chisel-shaped.

6. Do not sharpen the pencil over the drawing board.

7. Do not jab the legs of the dividers into the drawing board.

8. The joints of compass and divider should not be oiled.

9. The dividers should never be used as reamers or pincers.

10. Do not scrub a drawing all over with an eraser after finishing.

11. Always keep duster at hand to clean any dirt that might settle on the drawing equipment or the sheet.

12. Before leaving the place see that each piece in the instrument box is thoroughly cleaned.

2

Technical Lettering

INTRODUCTION

Graphical language must be accompanied by size description and instructive specifications in the form of figured notes and dimensions. The entire written information on the drawing is always in the form of lettering and not in handwriting. Lettering should be done on the drawing in such a manner that it may be read when the drawing is viewed from the bottom edge, except where it is used for dimensioning purposes.

Lettering on drawing should be legible, neat in appearance and correct in style. Single stroke letters have these qualifications, therefore, they are universally used for engineering working drawings. They should not be executed mechanically but should be made entirely freehand. Letters having all strokes of uniform thickness are classified as *Gothic*. The style of the letter, when the thickness of the strokes is such that it can be made with a single stroke of pencil, is called *Single Stroke Gothic*. The term *Single Stroke* does not imply that the letter is produced with a continuous movement of the pencil or pen, but that the letter is made of one or more stems or curves, each of which is made with a single stroke.

SINGLE STROKE VERTICAL LETTERS

An alphabet set of vertical capital letters is shown in Figs 2.1 and 2.2. To show each unit, every rectangle has been divided into smaller squares of one unit side. The direction of movement of the pencil point to mark the letter and different strokes to be executed are shown in Fig. 2.2. The general proportions of letters (7:5 and 6:5) are sufficiently accurate from the student's point of view to commence with. Horizontal strokes are made from left to right and vertical strokes from the top downwards.

Most of the strokes are natural and do not require memorizing, but the beginner must keep in mind that it is a decided mistake to practise lettering before he knows the proportions and order of strokes of the letter he/she is to execute. The beginners should consistently learn the forms of the letters by sketching them on a graph paper, taking different heights of letters, until they fully grasp the shapes and proportions of letters.

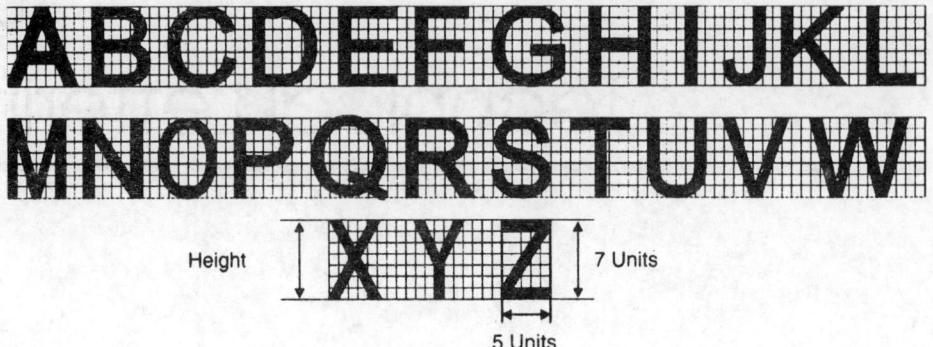

Height — 7 Units

5 Units

Fig. 2.1

For purposes of close analysis and practice, letters may be classified as:
1. Straight line combinations
2. Curved line combinations.

1. STRAIGHT LINE LETTERS (Fig. 2.2)

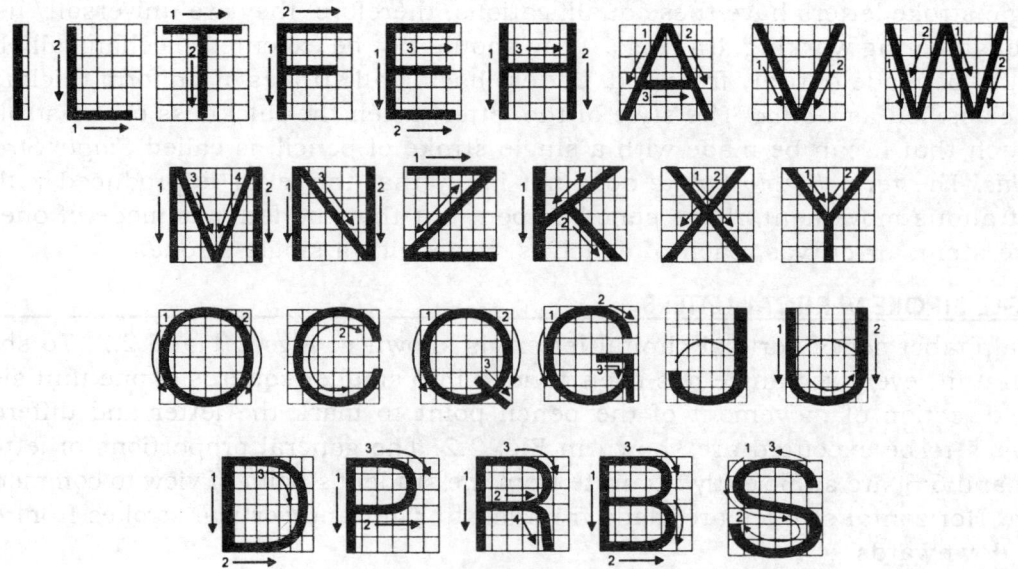

Fig. 2.2

ILT: The I and the vertical strokes of the letters L and T are drawn downward with a finger movement. The horizontal strokes are drawn from left to right. The normal width of the letter L is 4.5 unit as shown, but when it is followed in a word by a capital A, its width should be reduced to about 4 spaces to compensate for the large area between the letters.

FEH: Stoke 4 of the letter E is nearly three-fifths long as stroke 2, and is slightly above the mid-point. Stroke 3 of F is the same as stroke 4 of E. Stroke 3 of H is again slightly above the centre of its height.

AVW: Stroke 3 of A is at one-third the height of the letter from the base line. The letter W is 1.33 times the normal width of a letter and it is the widest letter in the alphabet.

MNZ: There is a decided advantage in drawing the parallel strokes of the letters M and N before drawing the diagonal strokes, as shown, strokes 3 and 4 of M, and strokes 2 and 3 of N should intersect in the base line. The strokes 3 and 4 of M intersect nearly two units above the base line.

KXY: Strokes 1 and 2 of K intersect at a point one-third the height of the letter from the base line. Stroke 3, extended, intersects stroke 2 at the top. The three strokes of Y intersect a little below mid-point. The strokes 1 and 2 of X intersect slightly above the centre.

2. CURVED LINE LETTERS (Fig. 2.2)

OCQG: The letters O, C, Q and G are formed with circles as bases. The letters O and Q are complete circles. The letters C and G are not complete circles and therefore, their width is slightly less than their height. Stroke 3 of Q is a radial line making an angle of 30° with a vertical. The horizontal stroke 5 of G begins at the centre of the circle and stroke 4 is vertical.

JUD: The letter J is a modification of U but is one-half spaces less in width. Stroke 3 of U is slightly elliptic and begins at a point one-third the height of the letter above the base line. The right side of D is circular.

PRB: Stroke 4 of P is slightly below the centre of height of the letter, while stroke 4 of R should be at mid-point and stroke 3 of B is slightly above mid-height.

S: The upper and lower portions of S are elliptic, the ellipses being tangent to a common vertical line on the left side. Compare S with the numerals 8 and 3.

SINGLE STROKE INCLINED CAPITAL LETTERS

The order and direction of the strokes and also the proportions of all the slant letters are exactly the same as those for vertical letters (Fig. 2.3). Inclined letters can be regarded as oblique projections of vertical letters. Inclined guidelines, made independently of the widths of the letters and spaces, will aid in getting a correct and uniform slant for inclined letters. The inclination is usually kept at 75°. The inclined direction lines should be drawn with a special lettering triangle of 75°. Essential requirements of this lettering are:

1. Keeping to a uniform slope.
2. Having the letters full and well shaped.
3. Keeping them close together.

Figure 2.3 shows letters printed in parallelograms of proportions 6:5, sufficiently correct from drawing point of view. The letters here too are grouped as straight line letters and curved line letters. These letters printed in 7:5 parallelograms, as recommended, are shown in Fig. 2.4.

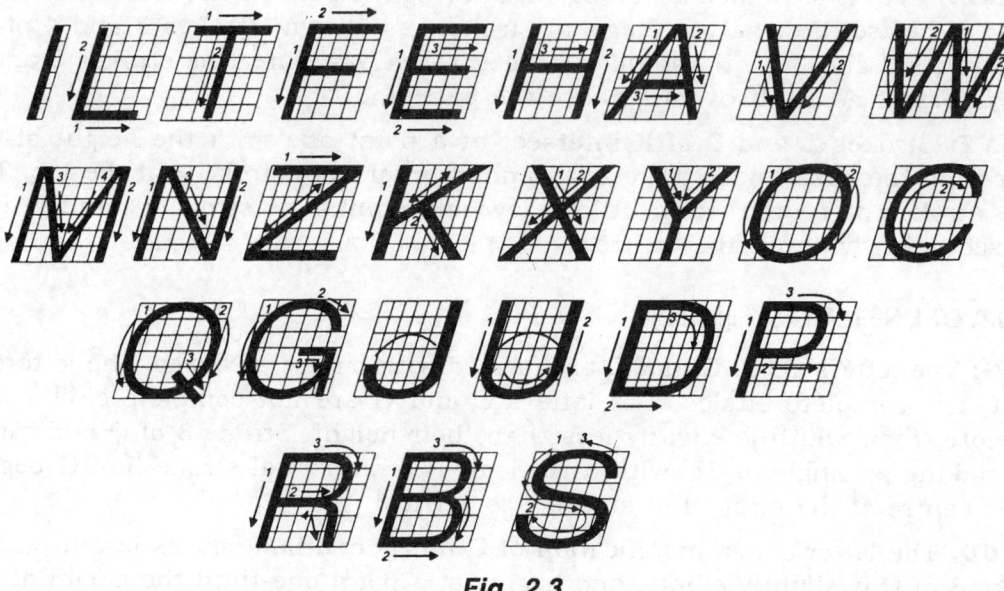

Fig. 2.3

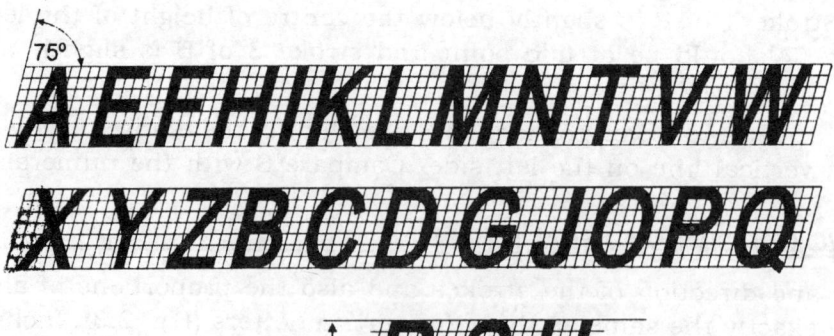

Fig. 2.4

SINGLE STROKE LOWERCASE LETTERS

These letters may be written in four guidelines. The body portion of letters is $\frac{2}{3}$ to $\frac{5}{7}$ of the height of related capitals. The ascenders extend to the cap line and descenders to the drop line (Fig. 2.5). Lowercase lettering may be vertical or inclined.

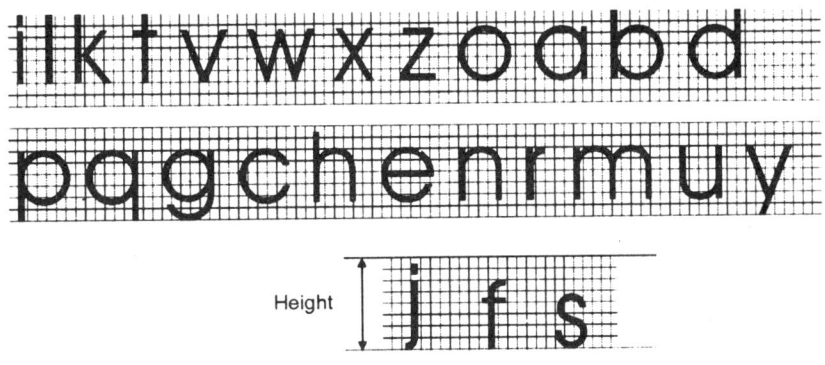

Fig. 2.5

VERTICAL LOWERCASE LETTERS

The letters **i, l, k** and **t:** All letters of this group are formed by straight lines.

The letters **o, s, v, w, x** and **z:** All of these letters are similar to the capitals.

The letters **a, b, d, p** and **q:** The bodies of the letters in this group are formed by letter o and they differ only in the position and length of the stem stroke.

The letter **g** is related to the letters **o** and **y.** Letter **e** is modified **o** and e is modification of **e.**

The letters **h, n, r** and **m:** The curve of the letter h is the upper portion of the letter **o.** The letter **n** differs from **h** in that the stem stroke extends only from waist-line to last line. The letter **r** is a portion of the letter **n.** The letter **m** consists of two modified **n**'s.

The letters **u** and **y:** The letter **u** is inverted **n.** The letter **y** is a practical combination of **u** and **g.**

The letters **j** and **f:** The portion of the letter **j** above the base line is letter **i.** The curve is same as of **y.** The width of curved portion of **f** is smaller than the other letters.

Also note that the body part of most of the letters in this proportion is a square of 4 units side and maximum height of letters is 6 units.

Figure 2.6 illustrates vertical lowercase letters. Body part of most of these letters are formed in rectangles of 5:4 whereas their height is 7 units. This proportion is to be preferred in practice.

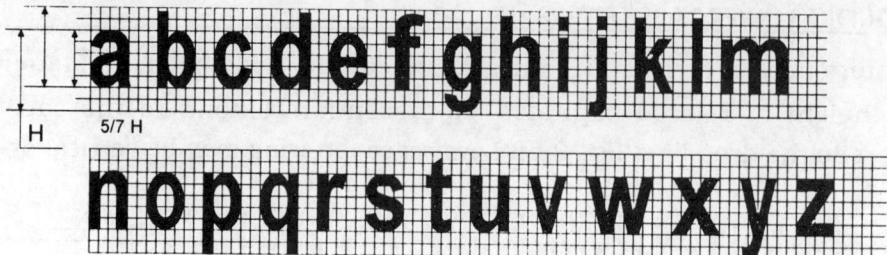

Fig. 2.6

INCLINED LOWERCASE LETTERS

The order and direction of the strokes and the proportion of all inclined lowercase letters are the same as for vertical lowercase letters. The lowercase inclined letters may be regarded, like the uppercase inclined letters, as oblique projections of vertical letters in which all of the circles in the vertical alphabet become ellipses in the inclined alphabet. As in inclined capital letters, all ellipses have their major axes sloping at an angle of 75° with the horizontal.

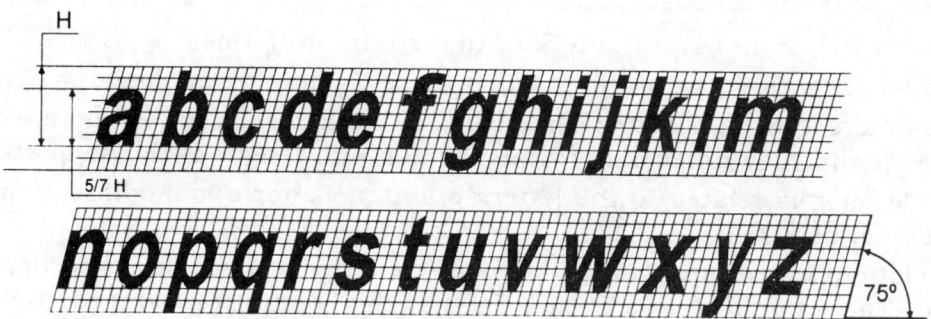

Fig. 2.7

Figure 2.7 illustrates inclined lowercase letters recommended. Body parts of most of these letters are formed in parallelograms of 5:4 whereas their height is units. See that body part of none of these letters is a circle.

VERTICAL NUMERALS

Both vertical and horizontal guidelines should be drawn for numerals too. This is particularly necessary for beginners. Since all values in engineering drawing are expressed by numerals, which should be perfectly legible, the student should make a careful study of their strokes and proportions.

All numerals except 1, in Fig. 2.8 are in rectangles of 7:4 and the numerals 3 and 8 are symmetrical about the centre. Numerals 6 and 9 have their loops up to exact centres of grid.

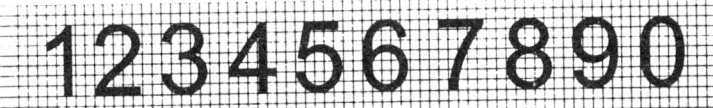

Fig. 2.8

In Fig. 2.9, all numerals except 1 are in rectangles of 6 units height and 5 units width. The numeral 1 is made with a single downward stroke.

The numeral 2 is made in two strokes, the first stroke, which passes through the centre of the grid, the second stroke at right angles to the end of first stroke.

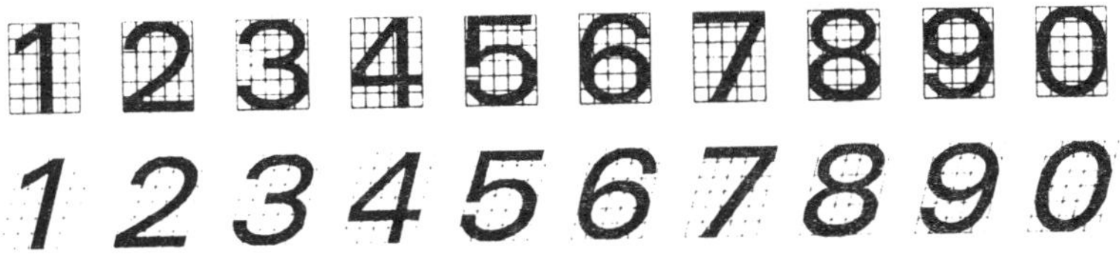

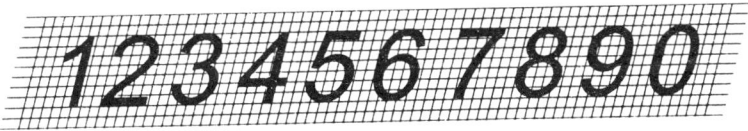

Fig. 2.9

The numeral 3 is of such a shape that it is nearly three-fourths of letter 8. The letter 4 is completed in three strokes. Stroke 3 is at one-fourth the height of the letter from the bottom.

The numerals 6 and 9 are elliptical. The numeral 9 is the same as 6 upside down. The loops in the numerals 6 and 9 are two-thirds as high as numerals.

The numeral 7 has its stroke 1 straight and its stroke 2 is slightly curved.

The numeral 8 is made up of a small ellipse on top of a large ellipse. The tangency of the two ellipses is slightly above the centre of grid, 0 is an ellipse.

The tops of the numerals 3, 5, 6 and 8 are narrower than the bottom to give them stability (Fig. 2.8).

INCLINED NUMERALS

Inclined numerals also are inclined at the same angle, i.e. 75° to the horizontal, as the inclined letter (Fig. 2.9). The inclined numerals may be regarded as oblique projection of vertical numerals, and the general proportion and stokes are the same.

Figure 2.10 illustrates vertical numerals printed in parallelograms of 7:4.

Fig. 2.10

ROMAN LETTERS

Specimens of vertical and inclined Roman letters are illustrated in Figs 2.11 and 2.12, respectively.

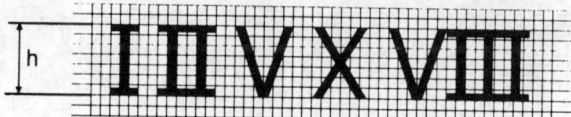

Fig. 2.11

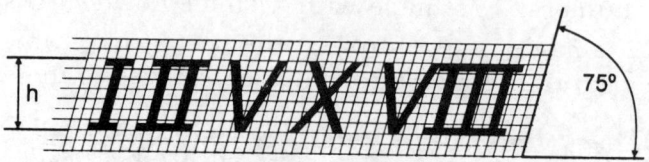

Fig. 2.12

ROMAN NUMBERS

Arabic	Roman	Arabic	Roman	Arabic	Roman
1	I	15	XV	100	C
2	II	16	XVI	101	CI
3	III	17	XVII	200	CC
4	IV	18	XVIII	300	CCC
5	V	19	XIV	400	CD
6	VI	20	XX	500	D
7	VII	21	XXI	600	DC
8	VIII	30	XXX	700	DCC
9	IX	40	XL	800	DCCC
10	X	50	L	900	CM
11	XI	60	LX	1000	M
12	XII	70	LXX	2000	MM
13	XIII	80	LXXX	3000	MMM
14	XIV	90	XC	4000	DM

GREEK ALPHABETS

α	β	γ	δ	ε	ζ	η	θ
Alpha	Beta	Gamma	Delta	Epsilon	Zeta	Eta	Theta
ι	κ	λ	μ	ν	ξ	o	π
Iota	Kappa	Lambda	Mu	Nu	Xi	Omicron	Pi
ρ	$\sigma\varsigma$	τ	υ	φ	χ	ψ	ω
Rho	Sigma	Tau	Upsilon	Phi	Chi	Psi	Omega
A	B	Γ	Δ	E	Z	H	Θ
Alpha	Beta	Gamma	Delta	Epsilon	Zeta	Eta	Theta
I	K	Λ	M	N	Ξ	O	Π
Iota	Kappa	Lambda	Mu	Nu	Xi	Omicron	Pi
P	Σ	T	Y	Φ	X	Ψ	Ω
Rho	Sigma	Tau	Upsilon	Phi	Chi	Psi	Omega

RUNNING LETTERS

abcdefghijklmnopqrstuvwxyz

CALIGRAPHY ART

Bhupal Nobles College of Pharmacy, Udaipur

The Times of India

New Delhi

"Simple Living High Thinking"

CALIGRAPHY LETTERS

𝔄 𝔅 ℭ 𝔇 𝔈 𝔉 𝔊 ℌ 𝔍 𝔍 𝔎
𝔏 𝔐 𝔑 𝔒 𝔓 𝔔 ℜ 𝔖 𝔗
𝔘 𝔙 𝔚 𝔛 𝔜 ℨ

𝔞 𝔟 𝔠 𝔡 𝔢 𝔣 𝔤 𝔥 𝔦 𝔧 𝔨
𝔩 𝔪 𝔫 𝔬 𝔭 𝔮 𝔯 𝔰 𝔱
𝔲 𝔳 𝔴 𝔵 𝔶 𝔷

0 1 2 3 4 5 6 7 8 9 ~ " " ?

COMPOSITION

Composition in lettering means the arrangement and spacing of words and lines with letters of approximate size and style. Make the letters broad but closely spaced. Open spacing is hard to read. Even spacing is essential as uneven spacing spoils the entire composition.

In combining letters into words, the spaces for the various combinations of letters are so arranged that they appear to be equal.

The key note of successful lettering is *uniformity*. Compact uniform lettering is an asset to any drawing. *Uniform height* is obtained by having each letter meet the top and bottom guidelines. *Uniform weight* by making all strokes of same thickness, *Uniform direction* by drawing and following direction lines, either vertical or inclined. *Uniform shade* by careful spacing. *Uniformity in strength* of lines can be acquired only by the skilful use of properly selected pencils.

In word spacing, the clear distance between them should be more than the height of the letters or they may be spaced by allowing room for the letter O between them. The space between sentences should be somewhat greater. The distance between the lines of lettering may vary from one-half the height of the capital to 1.5 times their height.

GENERAL PROCEDURE FOR LETTERING

The general procedure to make any type of lettering is suggested below.

1. Keeping in view the purpose of the lettering, decide the height of letters and draw horizontal guidelines, apart by height of letters and long enough to accommodate the printing.
2. Draw vertical or sloping guidelines as the case may be, on full length of horizontal guidelines, at random.
3. Keeping in view the shape and form or letters, plot lightly, all important points which are to serve as guides for different stokes to start and end.
4. Join these points in proper order by light pencil strokes.
5. When the shape of letters appear to be correct, and spaces balanced, fair out the letters and finish the work by removing reference guidelines.
6. Maintain proper distance between consecutive words in a sentence, different sentences and lines.

After a few letters are made, the pencil point will tend to become dull. To keep the lettering uniform the pencil point should be kept well sharp and the pencil should be continuously rotated in fingers while lettering.

LETTERING PENCILS

For ruling guideline a 3H or 4H pencil, well sharpened, is the best. The actual lettering should be done with a well sharpened H/HB pencil with a conical point. The pencil is first sharpened to a needle point and then the point is dulled slightly by marking on paper, rotating the pencil at the same time, to keep the point symmetrical. The pencil lead should be soft enough to produce jet-black letters, yet hard enough to prevent excessive wearing down of the point, and smearing of the graphite. The soft pencils containing more graphite, slide over the paper with less resistance and also produce a line dark enough to reproduce.

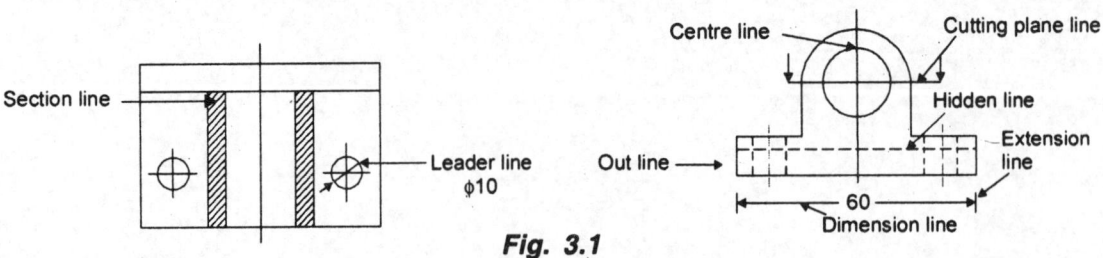

3

Dimensioning

DIMENSIONING

Dimensioning has an important place in drawing. Every drawing, either scale drawing or free hand drawing, must indicate length, breadth, height, size and locations of holes, slots, etc. Supply of this information on the drawing is called *dimensioning*.

There are two types of dimensions.

1. Function Dimensions

These are essential for the function of the product. It is also known as size dimension, e.g. length, breadth, height, depth, diameter, etc.

2. Location of Datum Dimensions

These are theoretically exact dimensions which locate a datum point, line or plane at which a feature should be within certain limits of size. It shows location or exact positions of various constructional details of the object.

NOTATIONS AND TERMS USED IN DIMENSIONING

1. Dimension Lines

Dimension line is a thin continuous line. It is terminated by arrowheads touching the outlines, extension lines or centre lines. There are thin full lines used to indicate the measurement. The amount of measurement is denoted by figures and should be placed near the middle and above, but clear of the dimension line (Fig. 3.1).

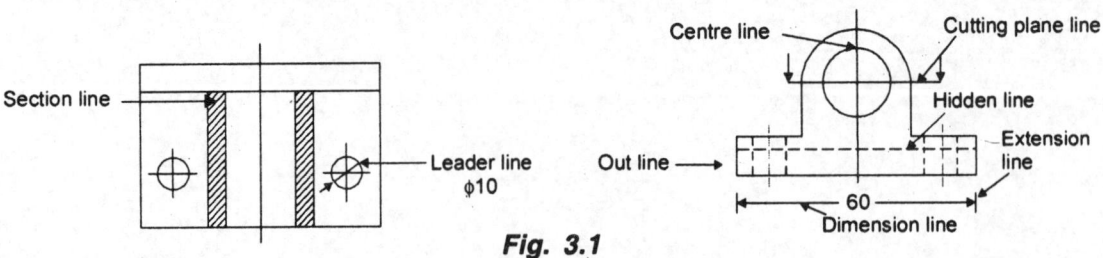

Fig. 3.1

2. Extension Line

These are thin full line extending beyond outlines and used when the dimension is to be placed outside the object. A gap of about 2 mm outside the outline of the object is kept and lines are extended 3 mm beyond the dimension lines (Fig. 3.1).

3. Leaders of Pointer Lines

These are the lines drawn from notes and figures to show where these apply. These are thin straight lines and terminated by arrowheads or dots. Leaders are drawn at any convenient angle, usually 30° or 45° or 60°. Leaders are never drawn vertical, horizontal or curved. Use of long leaders should be avoided. Figure 3.2 shows the correct and incorrect leaders.

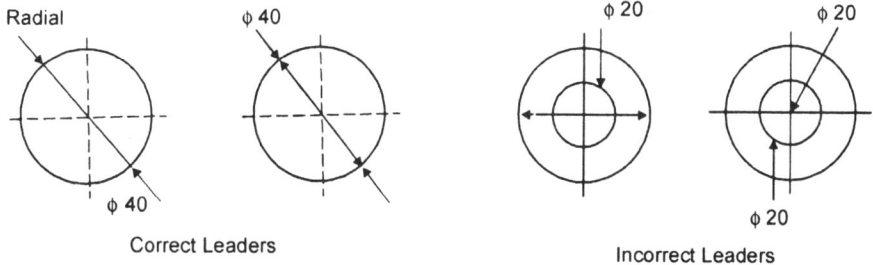

Fig. 3.2

When the space is not sufficient to draw the arrowheads from inside, they may be placed from outside as shown in Fig. 3.3. A dot may be used for replacing arrowhead. If the space is insufficient to give dimension, it may be written above the extended dimension line.

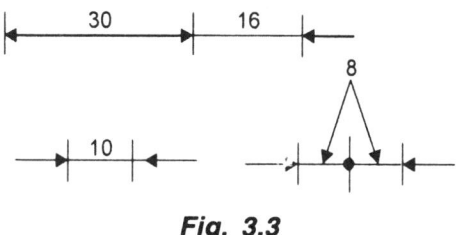

Fig. 3.3

4. Arrowheads

These are used to terminate the dimension lines. The length of arrowhead should be about three times its maximum width and normally it is 3 mm for small drawings and 4 to 5 mm for large drawings. The space in arrowheads should be filled in Fig. 3.4.

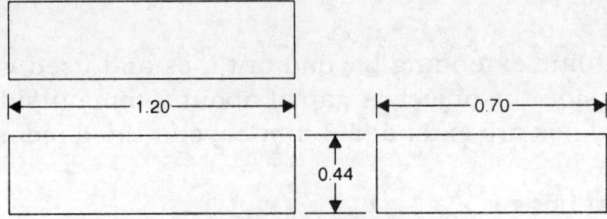

(a) Place dimensions between views

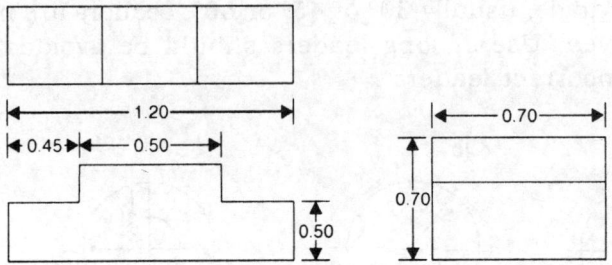

(b) Place smallest dimension nearest the view being dimensioned

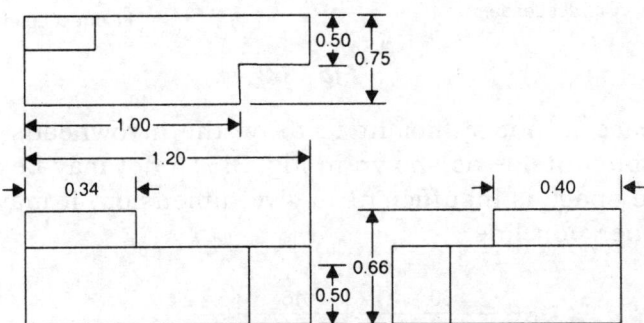

(c) Dimension the view that best shows

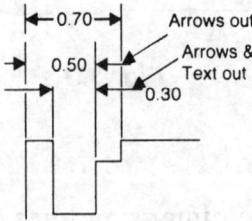

(d) Dimensions of the pipe

Fig. 3.4

Types of Lines

According to I.S.I., for general engineering drawing, following types of lines are used:

Type	Type of Line	Illustration	Uses
A.	Visible line/ continuous line		Out line, visible edges, surface boundaries of an object, margin line
B.	Continuous thin		Dimension lines, extension lines, section lines, pointer lines, construction lines, border lines
C.	Short break line		Short break lines or irregular boundaries lines
D.	Long break line		Long break lines, ruled line and short zigzag thin line
E.	Hidden line short dashes		Dotted or dashed or hidden lines
G.	Centre line		Centre line, locus line
H.	Cutting plane line		Cutting plane lines or section plane line
K.	Additional treatment		Indicate surface which are to receive additional treatment

Units of Dimensioning

As far as possible all dimensions should be given in millimeters, omitting the abbreviation mm. When it is not convenient to give dimensions in millimeters and another unit is used only the dimension figures are written and a footnote *all dimensions are in centimeters* is inserted at an appropriate place near the title block.

Symbols of Materials

(Sectional view of various materials)
Symbols of various materials are used to represent them by conventions as follows.

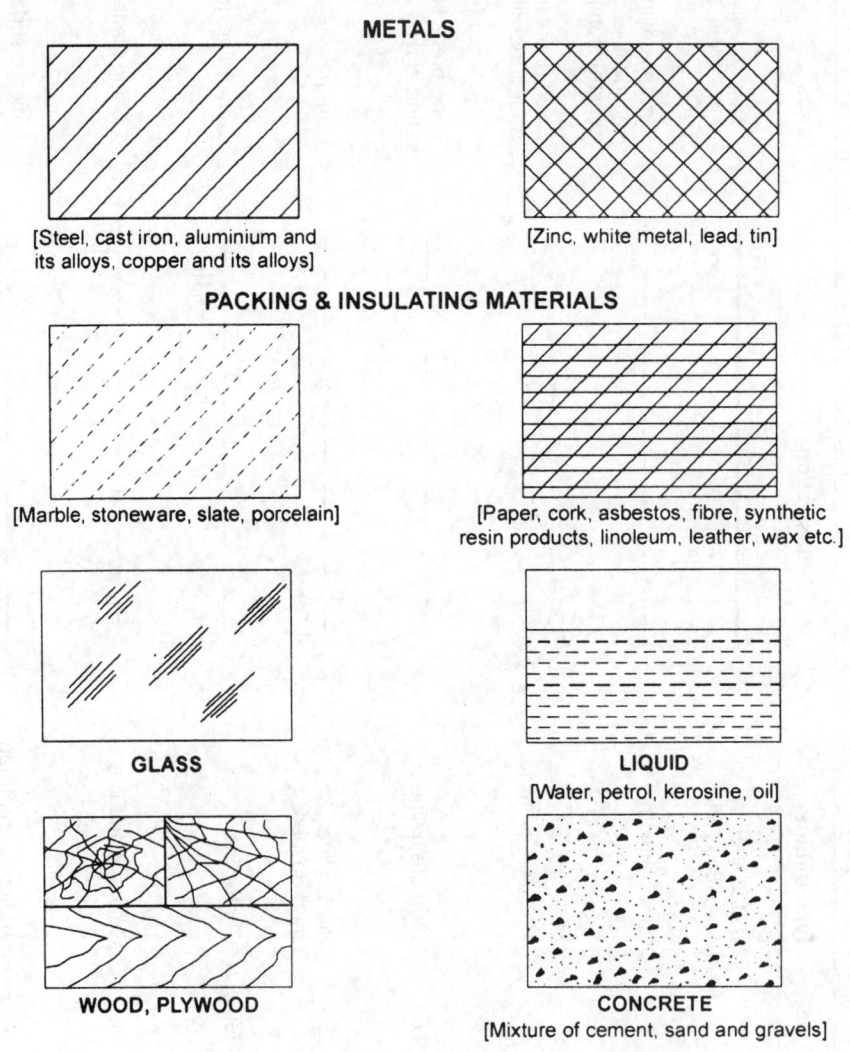

METALS

[Steel, cast iron, aluminium and its alloys, copper and its alloys]

[Zinc, white metal, lead, tin]

PACKING & INSULATING MATERIALS

[Marble, stoneware, slate, porcelain]

[Paper, cork, asbestos, fibre, synthetic resin products, linoleum, leather, wax etc.]

GLASS

LIQUID
[Water, petrol, kerosine, oil]

WOOD, PLYWOOD

CONCRETE
[Mixture of cement, sand and gravels]

Fig. 3.5: *Sectional view of various materials*

Rules for Dimensioning

1. Dimensioning should be completely done so as to avoid calculations, assumption of any dimension or direct measurement from the drawing.
2. Dimensions should be placed outside the views. However, they can be placed inside if they are more clear and easy to read inside.
3. Dimensions should be placed in the view where they show relevant features most clearly.
4. Every dimension must be given but dimension should not be repeated.
5. Dimension lines should be placed minimum 8 mm away from the outlines and from each other.
6. Dimension lines should not cross each other.
7. Dimensioning between the dotted lines should be avoided as far as possible.
8. Dimension line should not cross other lines in the drawing.
9. A centre line or the outline should not be used as a dimension line.
10. A centre line may be extended and used as an extension line.
11. If there are a number of dimensions, the shorter dimension should be nearer to the view.

Geometrical Constructions

4

BISECTING A LINE

Exercise

To bisect a given straight line.

- Let *AB* be the given line.
- From the point *A* and radius greater than half *AB*, draw arcs on both sides of *AB*.
- With point *B* and the same radius, draw arcs intersecting the previous arcs at *C* and *D*.
- Draw a line joining *C* and *D* and cutting *AB* at *E*.

    Then $AE = EB = \frac{1}{2} AB$.

- *CD* bisects *AB* at right angles (Fig. 4.1).

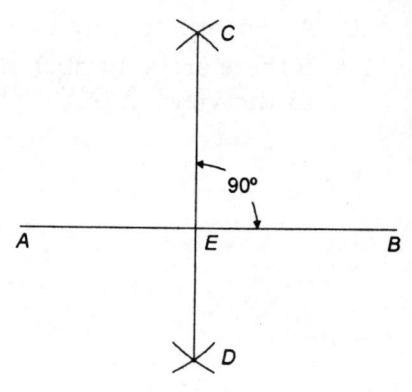

Fig. 4.1

Exercise

To draw a perpendicular to a given line from a point within it.

(a) When the point is near the middle of the line
- Let *AB* be the given line and *P* the point on it:
- From *P* as centre and any convenient radius R_1, draw an arc cutting *AB* at *C* and *D*.
- From any radius R_2 greater than R_1 and centres *C* and *D*, draw arcs intersecting each other at *O*.
- Draw a line joining *P* and *O* [Fig. 4.2 (a)].

(b) When the point is near an end of the line

- Let *AB* be the given line and *P* the point on it.
- From the point *P* as centre, draw an arc of any convenient radius cutting *AB* at *C*.
- From the same radius cut (from the arc) two equal divisions *CD* and *DE*.
- Again with the same radius and from centres *D* and *E*, draw arcs intersecting each other at *Q*.
- Draw a line joining *P* and *Q*.
- Then *PQ* is the required perpendicular [Fig. 4.2 (*b*)].

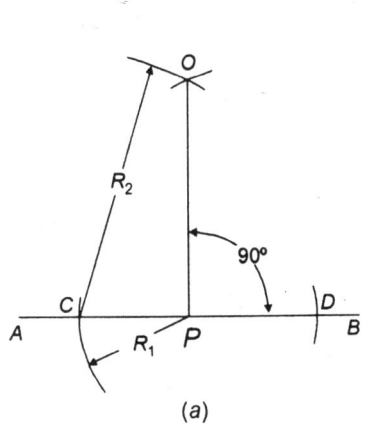

(a)

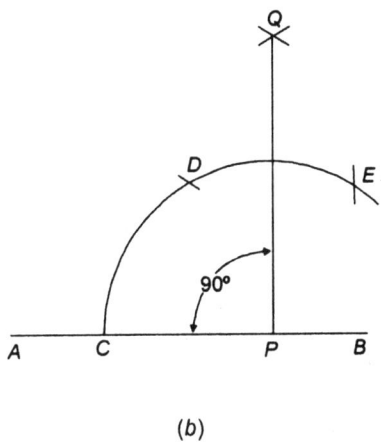

(b)

Fig. 4.2

Exercise

To draw a perpendicular to a given line from a point outside it (Fig. 4.3). When the point is nearer the centre than the end of the line.

- Let *AB* be the given line and *P* the point.
- From the point *P* and any convenient radius, draw an arc cutting *AB* at *C* and *D*.
- With any radius greater than half *CD* and centres *C* and *D*, draw the arcs intersecting each other at *E*.
- Draw a line joining *P* and *E* and cutting *AB* at *Q*.
- Then *PQ* is the required perpendicular.

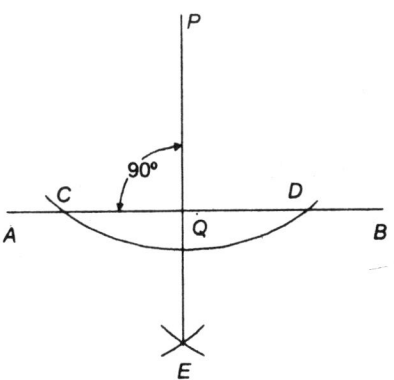

Fig. 4.3

TO DRAW PARALLEL LINES

Exercise

To draw a line through a given point, parallel to a given straight line.

- Let *AB* be the given line and *P* the point.
- From the point *P* and any convenient radius, draw an arc *CD* cutting *AB* at *E*.
- From the point *E* and the same radius, draw an arc cutting *AB* at *F*.
- From the point *E* and radius equal to *FP*, draw an arc to cut *CD* at *Q*.
- Draw a straight line through *P* and *Q*.
- Then this is the required line (Fig. 4.4).

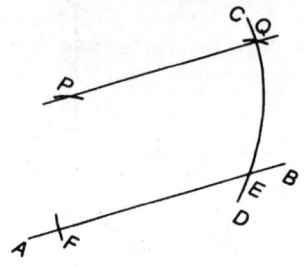

Fig. 4.4

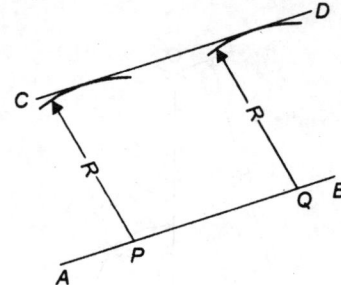

Fig. 4.5

Exercise

To draw a line parallel to and at a given distance from a given straight line.

- Let *AB* be the given line and *R* the given distance.
- Mark points *P* and *Q* on *AB*, as far apart as convenient.
- With *P* and *Q* as centres and radius equal to *R*, draw arcs on the same side of *AB* (Fig. 4.5).

TO DIVIDE A LINE

Exercise

To divide a given straight line into any number of equal parts.

- Let *AB* be the given line to be divided into, say, seven equal parts.
- Draw a line *AC* of any length inclined at some convenient angle to *AB* (preferably an acute angle).

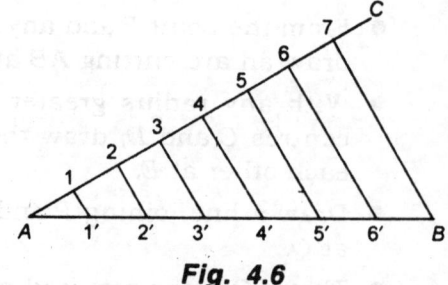

Fig. 4.6

- From *A* and along *AC*, cut-off with a divider seven equal divisions of any convenient length.
- Draw a line joining *B* and 7.
- With the aid of two set-squares, draw lines through 1, 2, 3, etc., parallel to *B7* intersecting *AB* at points 1', 2', 3', etc., thus dividing it into seven equal parts (Fig. 4.6).

TO BISECT AN ANGLE

Exercise

To bisect a given angle.

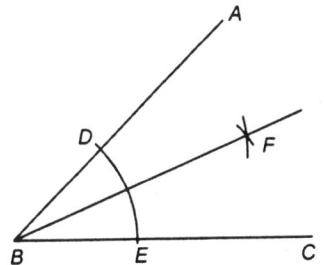 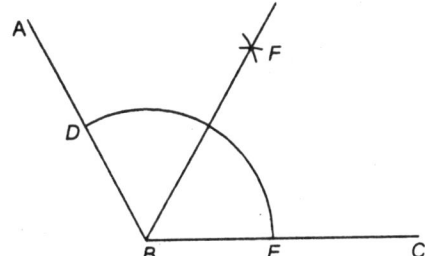

Fig. 4.7

- Let *ABC* be the given angle.
- From *B* as centre and any radius, draw an arc cutting *AB* at *D* and *BC* at *E*.
- From centres *D* and *E* and the same or any convenient radius, draw arcs intersecting each other at *F*.
- Draw a line joining B and *F*.
- *BF* bisects the angle *ABC* (Fig. 4.7).

Exercise

To draw a line inclined to a given line at an angle equal to a given angle.

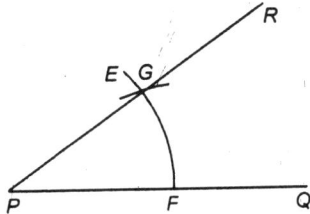 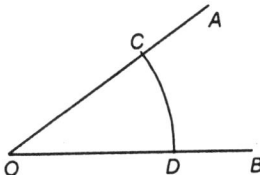

Fig. 4.8

- Let *PQ* be the given line and *AOB* the given angle.
- With *O* as centre and any radius, draw an arc cutting *OA* at *C* and *OB* at *D*.
- With the same radius and centre *P*, draw an arc *EF* cutting *PQ* at *F*.
- With *F* as centre and radius equal to *CD*, draw an arc cutting the arc *EF* at *G*.
- From *P*, draw a line passing through *G*.
- This is the required line (Fig. 4.8).

5

Construction of Scales

INTRODUCTION

It is not every time possible or convenient to make the linear dimensions on a drawing the same size as corresponding real dimensions on the object drawn. Drawings of very big objects, like a college building, must be drawn considerably smaller than the object, whereas details of small precision instruments, watches, etc. can be made larger than their real size. Large and small objects have to be drawn so that the drawings can be read and handled with convenience. If the linear dimensions of an object have to be enlarged or reduced for drawing purposes we resort to the use of scales which enable us to *enlarge (enlarging scale)* or *reduce (reducing scale)*. If the actual linear measurements of an object are shown in its drawing, the scale used is said to be a *full size scale.*

REPRESENTATIVE FRACTION

The ratio of the drawing to the object is called the representative fraction (abbreviated as RF)

$$RF = \frac{\text{Length of a line in the drawing}}{\text{Actual length of the line on the object}}$$

The dimensions in both numerator and denominator of the fraction must be in the same units. For example, if we wish to represent a dimension 2 metre by a line 4 cm long, it will be evident that the line when divided into 4 equal parts, each part will be 1 cm long and that this 1 cm length on the line represents 0.5 metre on the object. So we can say that we are using a scale or 1 cm to 0.5 metre.

$$RF = \frac{4 cm}{2 \times 100 \ cm} = \frac{1}{50}$$

We call this scale to be 1 : 50 without any mention of cm, metre or other linear units.

CONSTRUCTION OF SCALES ON DRAWINGS

When out of a set of recommended scales the required scale is not available, it has to be constructed on the drawing sheet. For constructing a scale, the following information is needed.

- The RF of the scale.
- The units it is to represent.
- The maximum length required to be measured.

Length of scale = RF × maximum length to be measured.

If the maximum length to be measured by a scale is not given, then we can take the length of the scale 15 cm to 30 cm.

Scales used in engineering practice are known as 'Draftsman Scales'. These scales are sold in sets of eight to twelve scales. The actual scale of the drawing should be written on the drawing sheet. The scale is mentioned by one of the ways given below.

1. 1 : 2 or 1/2 (RF)
2. Half/full size, etc.
3. 1 cm = 2 cm etc.

Table: Draughtsman's scales

Grade	Ratio		Grade	Ratio	
A	12 inches to a foot	1 : 1	M₁	100 cm to a metre	1 : 1
	6 inches to a foot	1 : 2		50 cm to metre	1 : 2
B	4 inches to a foot	1 : 3	M₂	40 cm to a metre	2 : 5
	2 inches to a foot	1 : 6		20 cm to metre	1 : 5
C	1.5 inches to a foot	1 : 8	M₃	10 cm to a metre	1 : 10
	3 inches to a foot	1 : 4		5 cm to metre	1 : 20
D	1 inch to a foot	1 : 12	M₄	2 cm to a metre	1 : 50
	0.5 inches to a foot	1 : 24		1 cm to metre	1 : 100
E	3/4 inches to a foot	1 : 16	M₅	1/2 cm to a metre	1 : 200
	3/8 inches to a foot	1 : 32		1/5 cm to metre	1 : 500
F	1/3 inches to a foot	1 : 36	M₆	1/3 cm to a metre	1 : 300
	1/6 inches to a foot	1 : 72		1/6 cm to metre	1 : 600
G	1/4 inches to a foot	1 : 48	M₇	1/4 cm to a metre	1 : 400
	1/8 inches to a foot	1 : 96		1/8 cm to metre	1 : 800
H	1/5 inches to a foot	1 : 60	M₈	1/10 cm to a metre	1 : 1000
	1/10 inches to a foot	1 : 120		1/20 cm to metre	1 : 2000

TYPES OF SCALES

Scales may be divided into the following six types.
1. Plain scales.
2. Diagonal scales.
3. Comparative scales.
4. Vernier scales.
5. Scale of chords.
6. Isometric scale.

PLAIN SCALES

Plain scale represents either two units or a unit and its subdivision (fractions). A plain scale consists of a line divided into suitable number of equal parts of units, the first of which is subdivided into small parts. For constructing a plain scale, we should:

- Calculate RF (if not given).
- Calculate length of the scale (L), using the formula L = RF × maximum length (rounded off to next higher whole number). If the maximum length to be measured is not known, use L = 15 to 30 cm.
- Draw a straight line of length L and divide it into a number of equal parts as required. Each part represents the larger unit.
- Place zero (0) at the end of the first main unit.
- Subdivide the division to the left of zero into subunits.
- Number the units towards right of (0) and the subunits towards its left.
- Write the names of the units and the subunits below the corresponding length of scale.
- Mention always the RF or the name of tile scale (e.g. 1 : 5) with the scale.

Exercise 1

Construct a scale of 1 centimetre = 1 metre to read metres and decimetres and long enough to measure up to 14 metre. Show a distance equal to 12.4 metre on it.

Solution

$$RF = \frac{1 \, cm}{1 \times 100 \, cm}$$

$$= \frac{1}{100}$$

Length of scale = RF × Maximum length to be measured

$$= \frac{1}{100} \times (14 \times 100) \text{ cm}$$

$$= 14 \text{ cm}$$

First of all, draw a line 14 cm long and divide it into 14 equal parts, each representing 1 m. Place zero at the end of the first division. Divide the first division (towards left of zero) into 10 equal parts, each representing 1 dm (decimetre) Complete the scale as shown in Fig. 5.1.

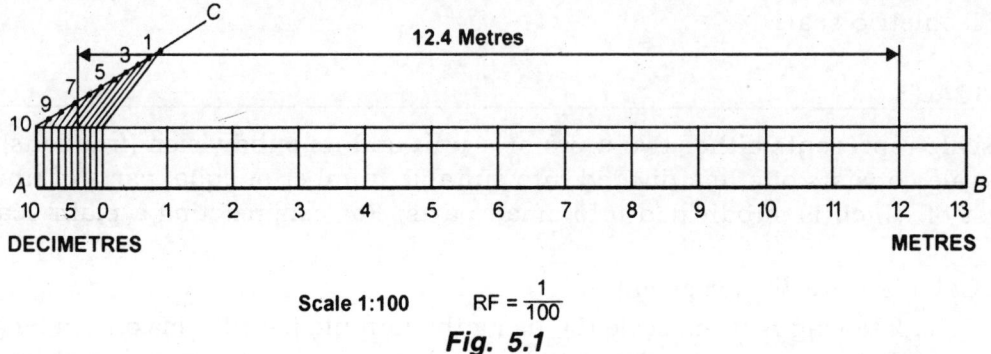

Scale 1:100   RF = $\frac{1}{100}$

Fig. 5.1

Exercise 2

Draw a scale of 1 : 50 (representative fraction 1/50) to show metres and decimetres, and long enough to measure up to 6 metre.

Solution

Length of scale = RF × maximum length to be measured

$$= \frac{1}{50} \times (6 \times 100) = 12 \text{ cm}$$

Draw a line *AB*, 12 cm long and divide it into six equal parts, each representing a metre. Name the divisions as is shown and subdivide the zero division into 10 equal parts, each representing a decimetre. Complete the scale as shown in Fig. 5.2.

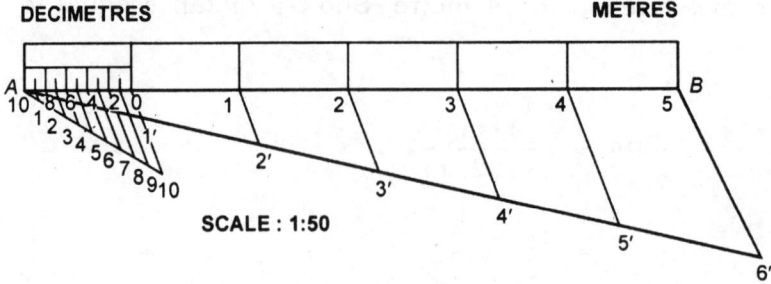

Fig. 5.2

Exercise 3

Draw a plain scale of representative fraction 1/40 or (1 cm = 0.4 m) to show metres and decimetres and long enough to measure up to 6 metre. Show a distance of 5 metre and 4 decimetre on it.

Solution

$$RF = \frac{1 \text{ cm}}{0.4 \times 100 \text{ cm}} = \frac{1}{40}$$

$$\text{Length of scale} = \frac{1}{40} \times \text{Maximum length to be measured}$$

$$= \frac{1}{40} \times (6 \times 100)$$

$$= 15 \text{ cm}$$

Draw a line AB, 15 cm long and divide it into six equal parts, each part representing a single metre.

Place 0 (zero) at the end of first main division and 1, 2 etc. at the end of subsequent divisions towards right of 0. Subdivide the zero division into 10 equal parts to represent single decimetre. Complete the scale and show the required distance as shown in Fig. 5.3.

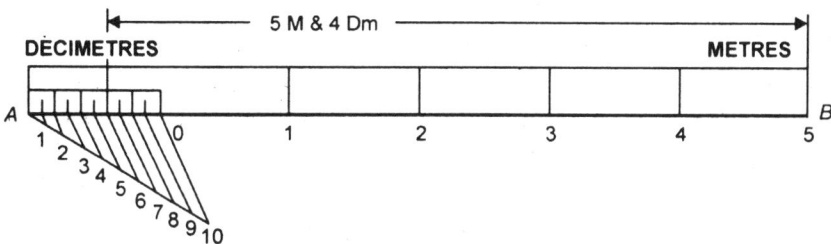

Fig. 5.3

Exercise 4

A rectangular plot 16 square kilometre is represented on a certain map by a similar rectangle of area 1 square centimetre. Draw a plain scale to show units of ten kilometre and single kilometre and long enough to read up to 60 km. Find RF of the scale. Also measure a distance of 53 kilometre on it.

Solution

$$\because \ 1 \text{ cm}^2 = 16 \text{ km}^2$$

$$\therefore \ 1 \text{ cm} = \sqrt{16} \text{ km} = 4 \text{ km}$$

$$RF = \frac{1\,cm}{4 \times 1000 \times 100\ cm} = \frac{1}{400,000}$$

Length of the scale = RF × maximum length to be measured

$$= \frac{1}{400,000} \times (60 \times 1000 \times 100)\,cm = 15\ cm$$

Therefore, draw a line 15 cm long and divide it into six equal parts, each representing 10 km. Subdivide the first part into 10 equal divisions each representing one km. Complete the scale as shown in Fig. 5.4.

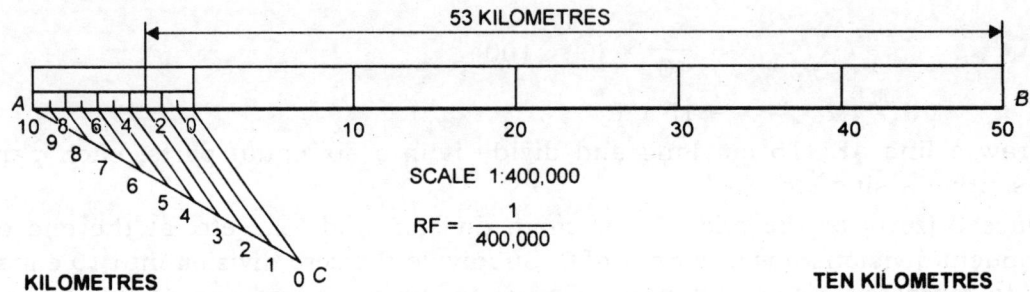

Fig. 5.4

Exercise 5

A rectangular plot of 25 square kilometres is represented on a certain map by a similar rectangle of area 1 centimetre. Draw a plain scale to show kilometres and long enough to measure unto 80 kilometres.

Solution

∵ 1 cm^2 = 25 km^2

∴ 1 cm = 5 km

$$\therefore \quad RF = \frac{1\ cm}{5 \times 1000 \times 100\ cm} = \frac{1}{500,000}$$

Length of scale = RF × Maximum length to be measured

$$= \frac{1}{500,000} \times (80 \times 1000 \times 100)\,cm$$

$$= 16\ cm$$

Draw a line 16 cm long and divide it into 8 equal parts, each representing 10 km. Divide the first part into 10 equal parts, each representing 1 km. Complete the scale as shown in Fig. 5.5.

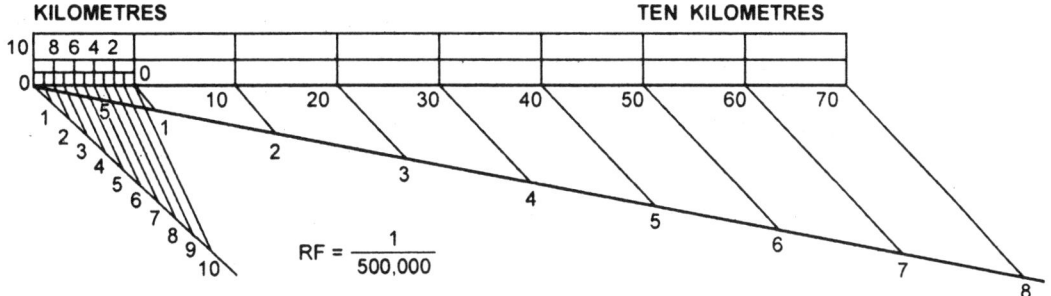

Fig. 5.5

Exercise 6

Construct a plain scale of 1 centimetre = 0.5 kilometre, to read kilometres and hectometres and long enough to measure up to 9 kilometres. Find its RF and measure a distance of 6 kilometres and 4 hectometres on the scale.

Solution

$$RF = \frac{1}{0.5 \times 1000 \times 100}$$

$$= \frac{1}{50,000}$$

$$\text{Length of scale} = \frac{1}{50,000} \times (9 \times 1000 \times 100) \text{ cm} = 18 \text{ cm}$$

Draw a line 18 cm long and divide it into 9 equal parts, each representing 1 km. Mark these main divisions and subdivide the first division into 10 equal parts, each representing 1 km and complete the scale as shown in Fig. 5.6.

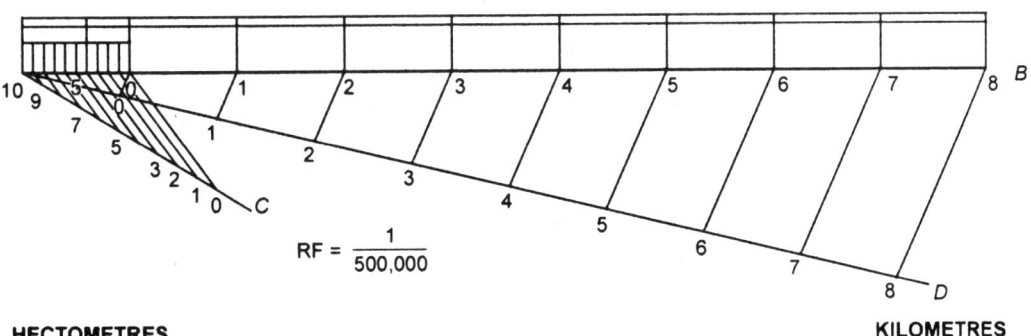

Fig. 5.6

Exercise 7

The distance between Ludhiana and Ambala Cantonment railway stations is 120 kilometres. A passenger train covers this distance in 4 hours. Construct a plain scale to measure time up to a single minute. The RF on the scale is 1/200,000. Indicate the distance covered by the train in 38 minutes on the scale.

Solution

As the length of scale is not given, therefore we assume it to be equal to 15 cm.

Since 1 cm = 200,000 cm, 15 cm length of scale will represent (200,000 × 15) cm = 30 km.

Average speed of the train 120/4 = 30 km.

Therefore, 30 kilometre distance is represented by 15 cm length of scale and is covered in 60 minutes.

Thus, draw a line 15 cm long and divide it into six equal parts. Each part then represents distance covered in 10 minutes and name the parts as shown. Subdivide the first part into 10 small divisions, each representing the distance covered in 1 minute. Complete the scale and indicate the distance covered by the train in 38 minutes as illustrated in Fig. 5.7.

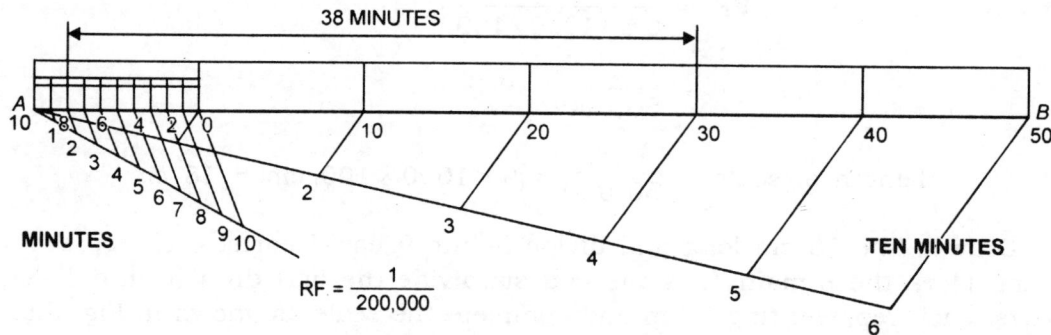

Fig. 5.7

Exercise 8

The distance between Delhi and Saharanpur is 180 kilometres. A passenger train covers this distance in 6 hours. Construct a plain scale to measure time up to a single minute. The representative fraction of the scale is 1/200,000. Indicate on it the distance covered by the train in 34 minutes.

Solution

$$RF = \frac{1}{200,000}$$

or   1 cm = 200,000 cm

                  1 cm = 2 km

$$\text{Speed of train} = \frac{180}{6} \text{ km/hour}$$

                  = 30 km/hr

                  = 0.5 km/minute

or 1 km in 2 minutes

Therefore   1 cm = 2 km

                  = 4 minute

1 cm line will represent 2 km distance which is covered in 4 minutes. Assume the maximum length of scale = 15 cm which will represent a distance of 30 km, covered in 60 minutes.

Divide 15 cm line into 6 equal parts, each part representing a distance of 5 km and time of 10 minutes. Subdivide the first part into 10 equal divisions. Each subdivision representing 1 minute and 0.5 km. Complete the scale as shown and indicate on it a distance of 17 km covered in 34 minutes (Fig. 5.8).

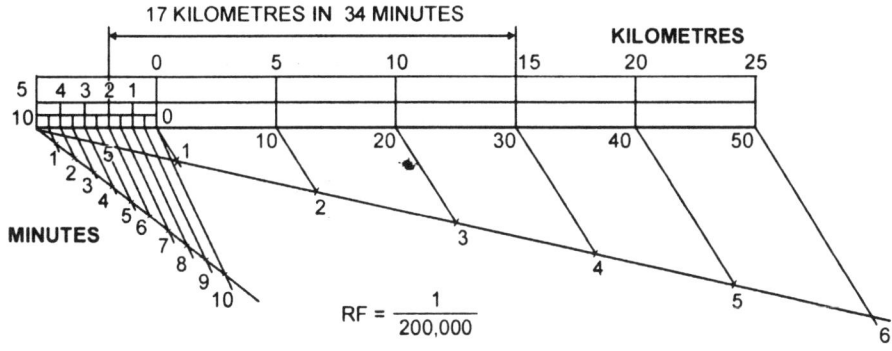

Fig. 5.8

DIAGONAL SCALES

Diagonal scale represents either three units or only one unit and its fractions up to second place of decimal point. It consists of a line divided into suitable number of equal parts, the first of which is subdivided into smallest parts by diagonals.

Subdivisions of a given short line can be obtained by the principle of diagonal division, as shown in Fig. 5.9. To divide a short line *AB* into ten equal divisions, e.g. 0.1 *AB*, 0.2 *AB*, 0.3 *AB* and so on, the procedure is as follows.

At *B*, draw a perpendicular *BC* to *AB* and step off 10 equal divisions of any convenient length along the perpendicular. Join *A* to *C*. Through the division points 1, 2, 3, 4, etc., draw lines 1–1′, 2–2′, 3–3′, 4–4′, etc. parallel to *AB*. As the triangles *ABC*, 9′9*C*, 8′8*C*, etc. are similar.

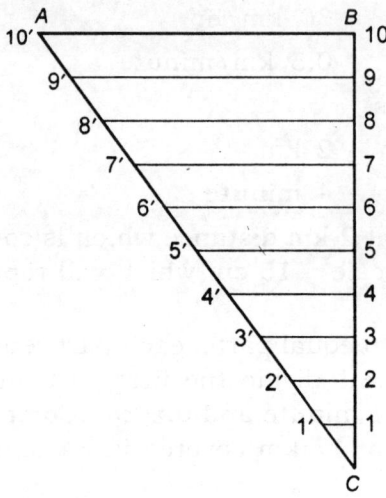

Fig. 5.9: *Diagonal divisions*

$$\because \quad \frac{C1}{CB} = \frac{11'}{AB}$$

$$\therefore \quad \frac{0.1 \times CB}{CB} = \frac{11'}{AB}$$

$$11' = 0.1 \times AB$$

Similarly as $\quad C1 = 0.1 \times BC$

$$C2 = 0.2 \times BC \text{ and so on.}$$

Excercise 9

A map 160 cm × 100 cm represents an area of 4000 km². Construct a diagonal scale to measure kilometres, hectometres and decametres. Find its RF. Indicate a distance of 6 kilometre, 5 hectometre and 7 decametre on this scale.

Solution

On this scale area of the map = (160 × 100) = 16,000 cm²

$\because$ 16,000 cm² map area represents an area or 4000 km²

$$\therefore \quad 1 \text{ cm}^2 = \frac{4,000}{16,000} \text{ km}^2$$

or $\qquad 1 \text{ cm} = \sqrt{\dfrac{4,000}{16,000}}$

$\qquad\qquad\qquad = 0.5 \text{ km}$

$\qquad RF = \dfrac{1}{0.5 \times 1000 \times 100}$

$\qquad\qquad = \dfrac{1}{50,000}$

Assume the length of scale to be 16 cm. The maximum distance which this scale can measure is 16 × 0.5 = 8 km. Therefore, draw a line AB 16 cm long and divide it into 8 equal parts, each part representing 1 km. Subdivide the first division (towards left of zero) into 10 equal parts, each showing single hectometre. Then, using the method of diagonal division subdivide each small division in 10 equal parts each representing 1 decametre. The distance of 6 kilometre, 5 hectometre and 7 decametre is indicated in Fig. 5.10.

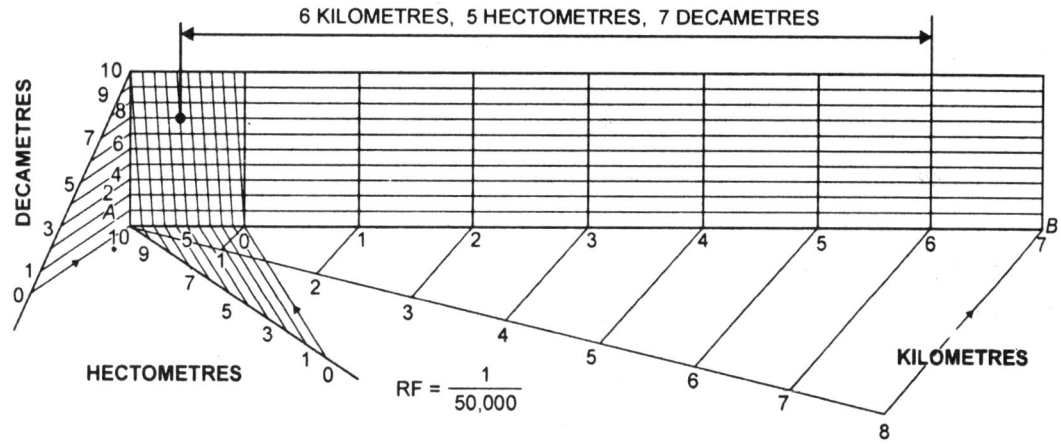

Fig. 5.10

Exercise 10

The distance between two stations is 600 kilometres. It is represented on a railway map by a line 15 cm long. Construct a diagonal scale to measure up to kilometres and find its RF. Indicate a distance of 346 km on the map.

Solution

$\qquad RF = \dfrac{15 \text{ cm}}{(600 \times 1000 \times 100) \text{ cm}}$

$$= \frac{1}{4,000,000}$$

Draw a line *AB* 15 cm long and divide it into six equal parts, each representing 100 km. Subdivide the first part into 10 equal divisions, each representing 10 km. Divide the first of these divisions by the method of diagonal division into 10 equal parts to represent single km. Complete the scale as illustrated in the Fig. 5.11. The distance of 346 km is indicated on the scale.

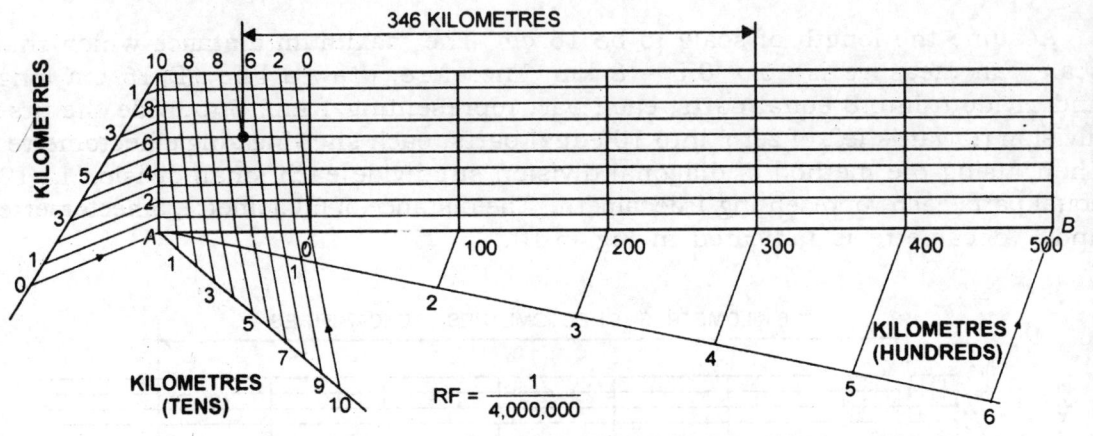

Fig. 5.11

Exercise 11

Construct a diagonal scale of 1 : 50 to show metres, decimetres and centimetres and long enough to measure up to 6 metres. Indicate on the scale a distance of 4 metres, 5 decametres and 4 centimetres.

Solution

$$RF = \frac{1}{50}$$

$$\text{Length of scale} = \frac{1}{50} \times (6 \times 100)$$

$$= 12 \text{ cm}$$

Draw a line *AB*, 12 cm long and divide it into 6 equal parts, each representing 1 metre. Divide the zero division into 10 equal parts. each representing 1 decametre. By diagonal division, further, divide each dm division into 10 parts each small part representing a centimetre; as shown in the Fig. 5.12. The distance of 4 m, 5 dm and 4 cm is indicated on the scale.

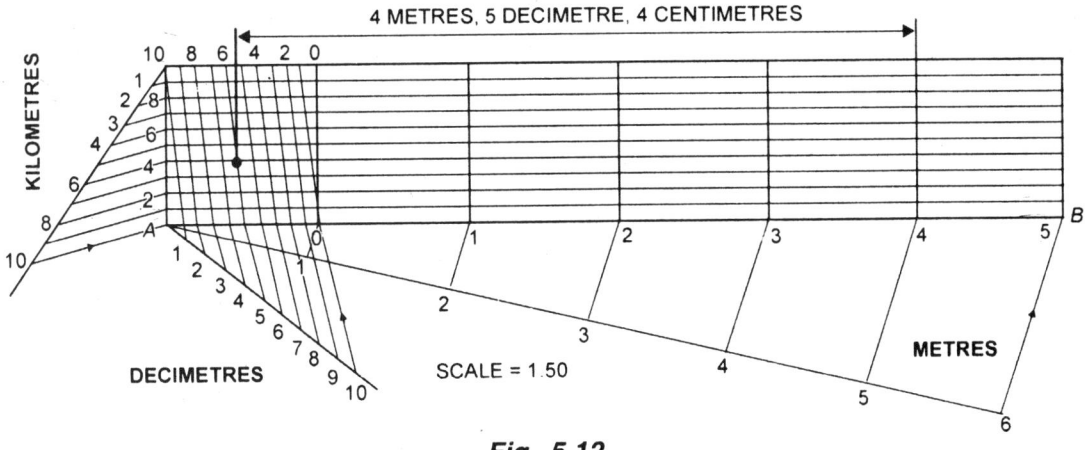

Fig. 5.12

Exercise 12

The distance between Ludhiana and Chandigarh is 100 kilometres and is represented on a certain road map by a line 2.5 cm long. Find the RF of the scale of the map and draw its diagonal scale showing single kilometre and long enough to measure up to 600 kilometres. Indicate on the scale the distance 573 kilometres.

Solution

$$RF = \frac{2.5}{100 \times 1000 \times 100} = \frac{1}{4,000,000}$$

Length of scale = RF × maximum distance which is to be measured

$$= \frac{1}{4,000,000} \times 600 \times 1000 \times 100 = 15 \text{ cm}$$

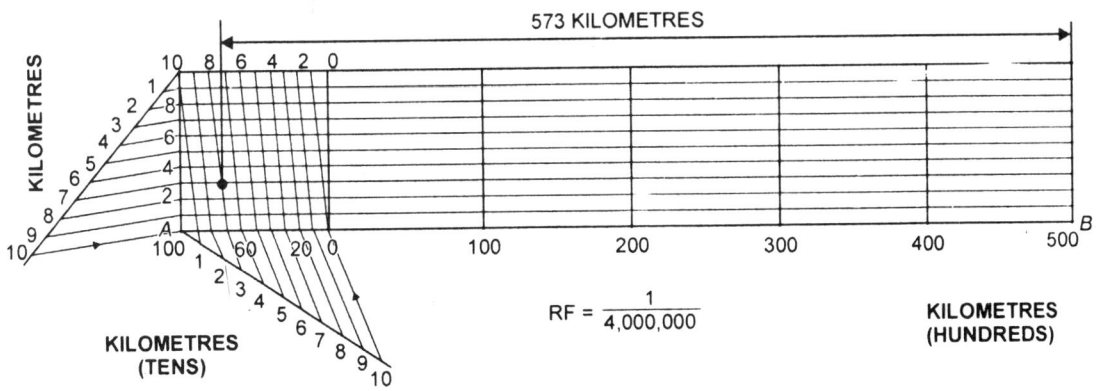

Fig. 5.13

Draw a line 15 cm long and divide it into six equal parts, each representing 100 km. Subdivide the first division (to the left of zero) into 10 equal parts, each representing 10 km. Then, divide each small division into 10 equal subdivisions using the principle of diagonal division. Complete the construction as shown in Fig. 5.13. Distance of 573 km is indicated on the scale.

Exercise 13

A rectangular plot of land area 0.45 hectare is represented on a map by a similar rectangle of 5 square centimetre. Calculate the RF of the scale of the map. Also draw a scale to read up to single metre from the map. The scale should be long enough to measure 400 metres.

Solution

$$\text{We know that 1 hectare} = 10,000 \text{ sq metres}$$

$$\therefore \quad 0.45 \text{ hectare} = 0.45 \times 10,000 = 4500 \text{ m}^2$$

$$= 4500 \times 10^4 \text{ cm}^2$$

$$\therefore \; 5 \text{ cm}^2 \text{ on map represents} = 4500 \times 10^4 \text{ cm}^2 \text{ on land}$$

$$\therefore \; 1 \text{ cm}^2 \text{ on map represents} = 900 \times 10^4 \text{ cm}^2 \text{ on land}$$

$$\therefore \quad 1 \text{ cm on map represents} = \sqrt{900} \times 10^2 \text{ cm}$$

$$= 30 \times 10^2 \text{ cm}$$

$$\therefore \qquad \text{RF of the scale} = \frac{1}{3,000}$$

$$\text{Length of the scale} = \text{RF} \times \text{max. length to be measured}$$

$$= \frac{1}{3,000} \times (400 \times 100) = 13.33 \text{ cm}$$

Draw a line 13.33 cm long and divide it into 4 equal parts, each part representing 100 metres. Divide the first (zero) division into 10 equal parts, each representing 10 metres. Further subdivide each such division by diagonal division into 10 equal parts, each smallest division representing single metre. Complete the diagonal scale as shown in Fig. 5.14.

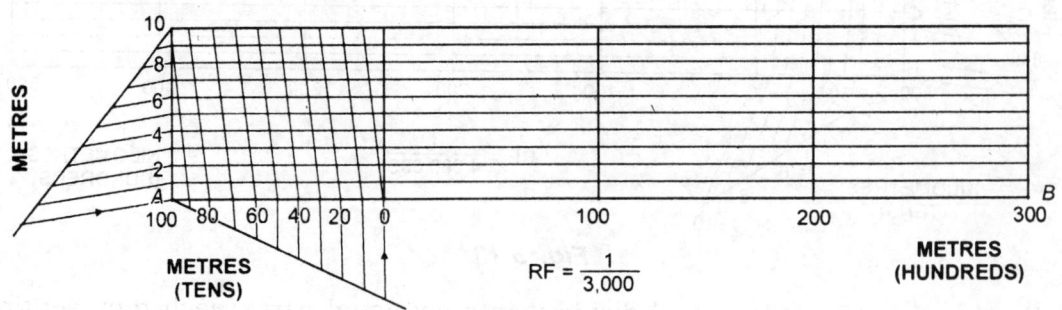

Fig. 5.14

Exercise 14

Draw a full size diagonal scale to read metres, decimetres and centimetres when its RF is 1/60 and long enough to read 9 metres.

Solution

$$RF = \frac{1}{60}$$

Length of scale = RF × max. length to be measured

$$= \frac{1}{60} \times (9 \times 100) = 15 \text{ cm}$$

Draw a line 15 cm long and divide it into 9 equal parts, each part representing a metre. Divide the first (zero) division into 10 equal parts, each part representing a decimetre. Then subdivide, each smallest part representing a centimetre. Complete the scale as illustrated in Fig. 5.15.

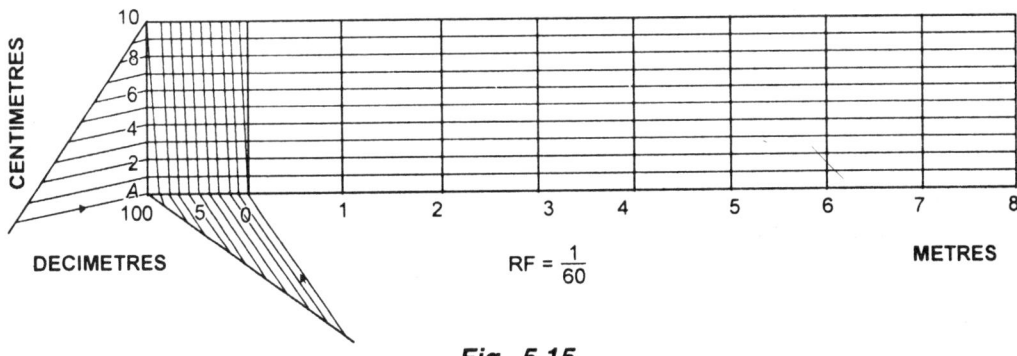

Fig. 5.15

Exercise 15

On a plane, a line 22 cm long represents a distance of 440 metres. Draw a diagonal scale for the plan to read up to single metre. Measure and mark a distance of 287 metres on the scale.

Solution

Now   22 cm = 440 metres

$$= 440 \times 100 \text{ cm}$$

∴ $$RF = \frac{22 \text{ cm}}{(440 \times 100) \text{ cm}} = \frac{1}{2000}$$

Assuming the max. length to be measured = 300 m

∴ Length of the scale

$$= \frac{1}{2000} \times (300 \times 100) \text{ cm} = 15 \text{ cm}$$

Thus draw a line 15 cm long and divide it into four equal parts, each representing 100 m. Divide the zero division into 10 equal parts, each representing 10 metres. Then subdivide each small division into 10 equal parts, by diagonal division, each equal part, each smallest division representing single metre. Complete the scale as shown in Fig. 5.16.

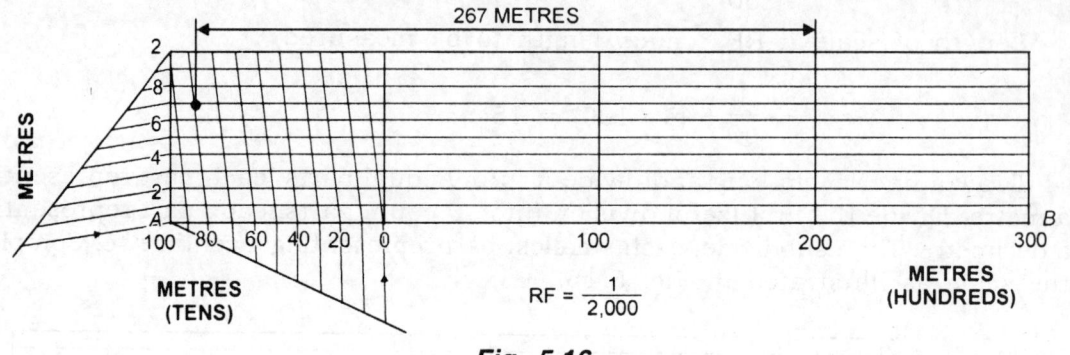

Fig. 5.16

COMPARATIVE OR CORRESPONDING SCALES

Scales having same RF but graduated to read different units are called *Comparative* or *Corresponding Scales*. These scales may be plain scales or diagonal scales and may be constructed one above the other or separately.

Exercise 16

On a railway map a scale of miles is shown. On measuring from this scale, a distance of 36 miles between two stations is represented by a line 6 cm long. Construct a plain scale to read miles and long enough to read up to 90 miles. Also construct a comparative scale attached to it, to read kilometres and read a distance up to 145 kilometres (1 mile = 1609 m).

Solution

1. Scale of miles:

$$\text{Length of scale} = \frac{6}{36} \times 90 = 15 \text{ cm}$$

Draw a line 15 cm long and construct a plan scale to show miles.

$$RF = \frac{6}{36 \times 1609 \times 100} = \frac{1}{96500}$$

2. Scale of kilometres:

$$\text{Length of scale} = \frac{1}{9654600} \times 145 \times 1000 \times 100 = 15.018 \text{ cm.}$$

Construct the plain scale 15.018 cm long, above the scale of miles, to read kilometres, as shown in Fig. 5.17.

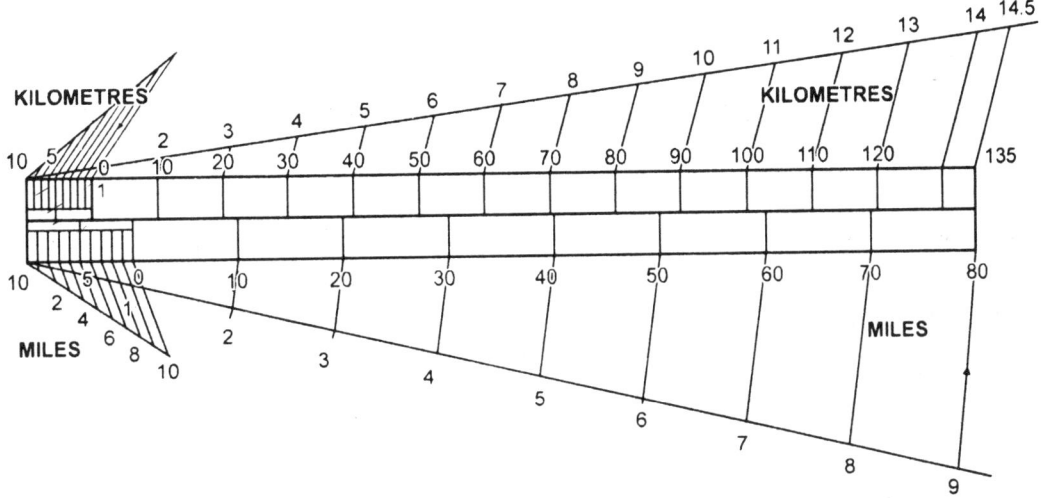

Fig. 5.17

VERNIER SCALE

Vernier scales are used to measure very small units with great accuracy. These scales can be said to be the modified form of diagonal scale. A vernier scale can be said to be the modified form of diagonal scale. A vernier scale consists of a primary scale and a vernier scale. The primary scale is a plain scale. For subdividing the smallest division on the primary scale, a vernier, which slides on the scale, is used. The gradations on the vernier are, therefore, derived from those on the primary scale.

Principle of Vernier

If a line representing units of measurement by dividing into n equal parts, each part will represent $\dfrac{n}{n} = 1$ unit whereas if a line equal to $n + 1$ of these units is taken and divided into n equal parts, each such part will be equal to $\dfrac{n+1}{n} = 1 + \dfrac{1}{n}$ units. Similarly, the difference between two parts from each will be equal to $\dfrac{n+1}{n} - \dfrac{n}{n} = \dfrac{1}{n}$ units. Similarly, the difference between two parts from each will be $\dfrac{2}{n}$ units.

Exercise 17

Construct a vernier scale, RF = $\dfrac{1}{40}$ of metres to show centimetres and long enough to read up to 6 metres. Indicate a length of 4.66 m on the scale.

Solution

$$\text{Length of scale} = \text{RF} \times \text{maximum distance which can be measured}$$

$$= \frac{1}{40} \times (6 \times 100) = 15 \text{ cm}$$

Therefore, draw a line 15 cm long and divide it into 6 equal parts to show metres. Subdivide each of these parts into 10 equal parts to show decimetres.

To construct a vernier, take 11 parts of one cm length on the left side of the zero division, and divide it into 10 equal parts, each representing a length of 1.1 dm or 11 cm and complete the scale as shown in Fig. 5.18. The length 4.66 m is indicated on the scale.

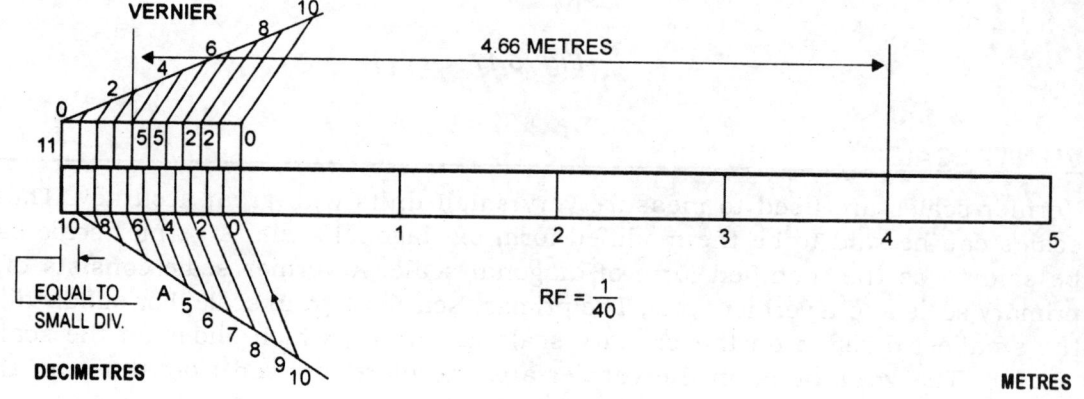

Fig. 5.18

Exercise 18

Draw a vernier scale of miles to show furlongs when 7 miles are represented by 1.4 inch and measure a distance of 25 mile 7 furlong on the scale.

Solution (Fig. 5.19)

$$\text{RF} = \frac{1.4 \text{ inch}}{(7 \times 1760 \times 3 \times 12) \text{ inch}}$$

$$= \frac{1}{316800}$$

Assuming the maximum length to be measured on the scale to be 35 miles. Length of the scale = RF × max. length to be measured

$$= \frac{1}{316800} \times (36 \times 1760 \times 3 \times 12) = 7 \text{ inch.}$$

Therefore, draw a line 7 inch long and divide it in 35 equal parts, each representing a single mile. Place zero at the end of the first eight divisions of the main scale from left. Place zero of the vernier vertically above the zero of the main scale.

Then take 9 parts of the main scale on the vernier and divide the length covered by them into eight equal parts, each part representing 1 mile 1 furlong. Number the parts as shown in the figure below.

To measure 25 mile 7 furlong, take 18 miles on the main scale and seven divisions of the vernier which represents 7 mile and 7 furlong, which make the total equal to 25 mile and 7 furlong as marked on the scale.

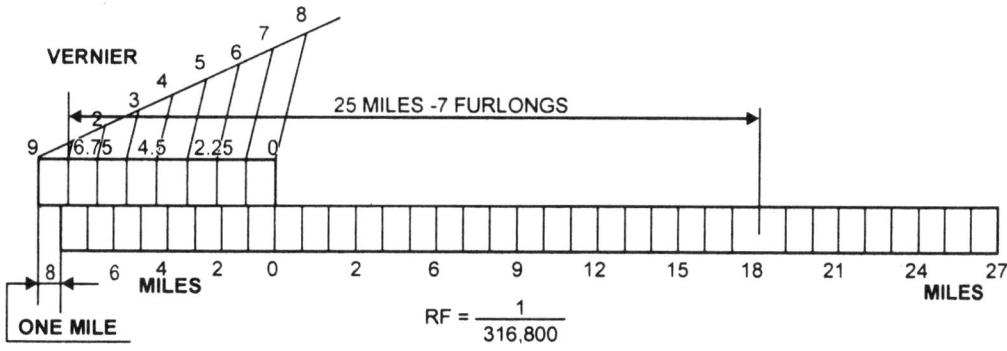

Fig. 5.19

6

Projection

When straight lines are drawn from various points on the contour of an object to meet a plane, the object is called to be projected on that plane. By joining the various points in correct sequence, the figure which formed is called a projection of the object and the lines are called **projectors**.

ORTHOGRAPHIC PROJECTION

Orthographic projection is formed when projectors are parallel to each other and also perpendicular to the plane. Orthographic projection may produce an image of a specified, imaginary object as viewed from any direction of space. It is distinguished by parallel projectors from the imaged object and which intersect a plane of projection at right angles. Orthographic projection shows the object as it looks from the front, right, left, top, bottom or back and are typically positioned relative to each other according to the rules of either first angle or third angle projection.

Vertical Plane

When we look at an object from a theoretically infinite distance, the rays of sight from our eyes will be parallel to one another and perpendicular to the front surface. When these rays are extended to meet perpendicularly and exactly, the same picture will be formed which is known as **vertical plane.**

Now further assume that a horizontal plane (HP) is hinged to the vertical plane so that the object will be in front of the vertical plane (VP) and above the horizontal plane. When we will look at the object from above, the view of the top surface of the object will be exactly the same as in Fig. 6.2. It shows only width and length of the object.

The horizontal plane when turned and brought in line with the VP is shown by dotted lines. The two projections can be shown on a flat surface in correct relationship with each other as shown in Fig. 6.1.

The projection on the vertical plane is called the front view or elevation. The projection on the horizontal plane is called the top view or plan.

VP and HP are not sufficient to describe an object completely. Therefore, an auxiliary vertical plane (AVP) is imagined to be placed at right angles to both AV and HP of the projections. The projection on this plane is marked by S and is the view of side surface of the object and is called a side view, end view, side elevation or end elevation. When AVP is rotated towards right side, the projection obtained as shown in Fig. 6.4.

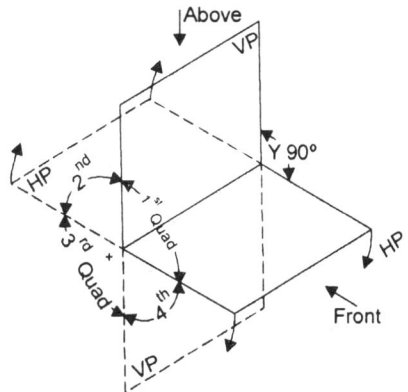

Fig. 6.1: *Four quadrants*

Besides the front view (VP), top view (HP) and side view (AVP) there are some possibilities to draw some more views, e.g. right side view, back view and bottom view as shown in Fig. 6.4 (*a*), (*b*), (*c*).

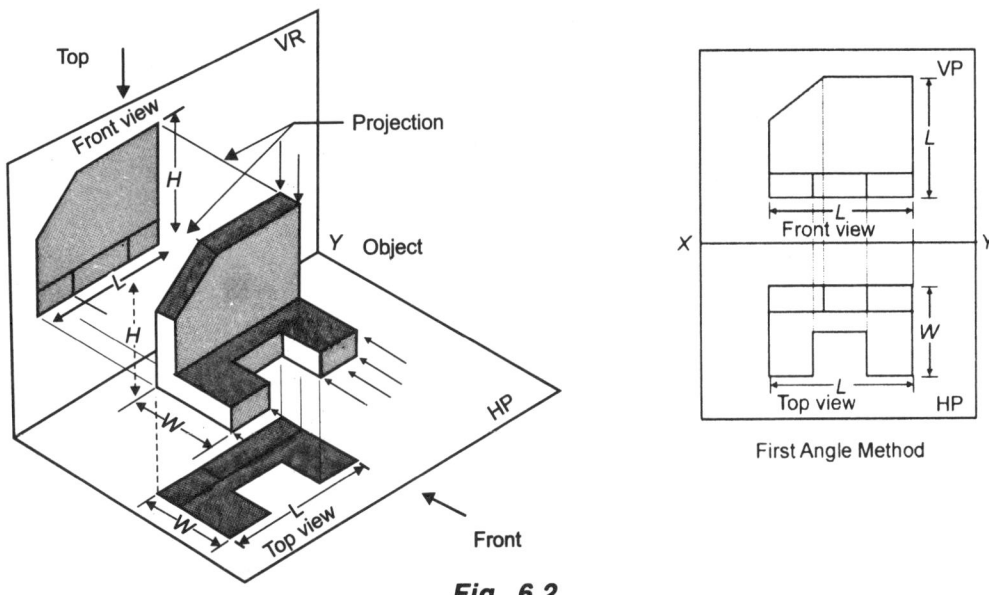

Fig. 6.2

Generally out of the six views only three views, i.e. front view, top view and a side view is necessary to describe an object completely.

Method of First Angle Projection

The ISO standard considers a projection on the opposite direction like X-ray/radiography. According to this the top view is under the front view, the right view is at the left of the front view. This method is used in Europe and Asia. When the two principal planes of projection are extended beyond their lines of meeting, they form four quadrants (Fig. 6.1). When we assume that the object is to be placed in front of VP and above the HP is known as first quadrant and the method of projection is known as first angle method of projection. In this method the top view comes below the front view and the view of the object as seen from the left side is placed to the right side of the front view and *vice versa* and is represented by the symbol shown in Fig. 6.3(a) and projections are shown in Fig. 6.4(b).

Method of Third Angle Projection

The American standard places the left view on the left and the top view on the top. This method is used in the United States and Canada. In this method the planes of projection are assumed to be transparent and objects assumed to be placed in the third quadrant. When the observer views the object from the front, the rays of the sight intersect the VP and front view will be formed by joining the points of intersection in correct sequence. The top view will be obtained by looking at the object from above. When these two planes are brought in line with each other, the views will be as seen in Fig. 6.5(a, b). The side view is obtained by projecting on an AVP, placed perpendicular to both the HP and the VP and between the observer and the object. The top view in this case comes above the front view and side view towards left side of the front view and is represented by the symbol [Fig. 6.3 (b)].

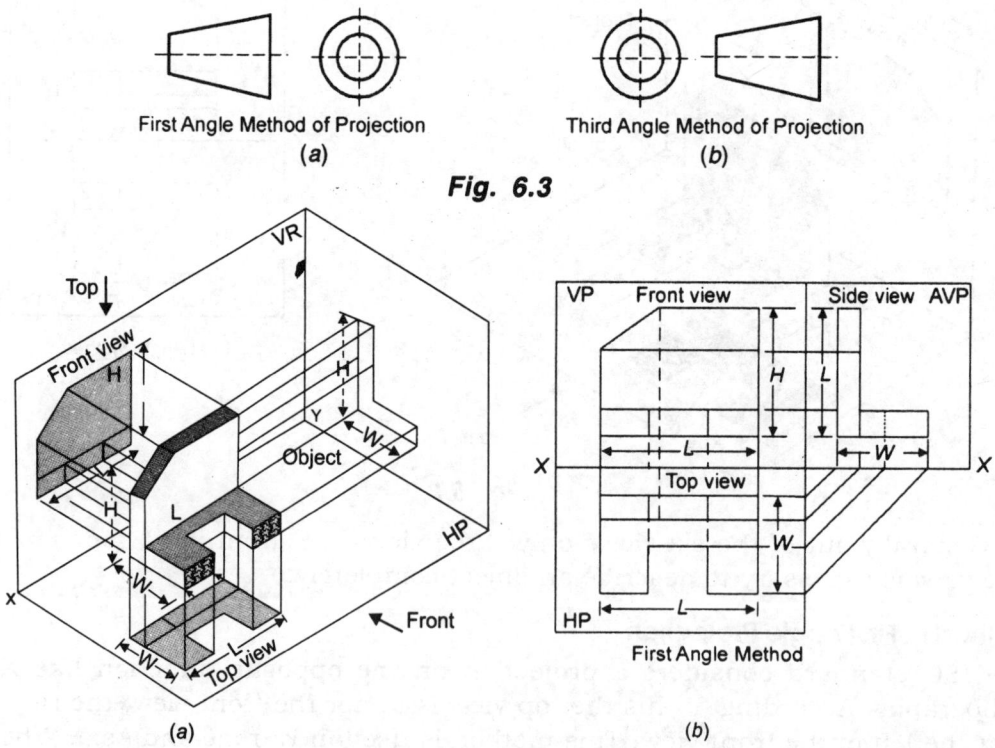

First Angle Method of Projection
(a)

Third Angle Method of Projection
(b)

Fig. 6.3

(a)

First Angle Method

(b)

Fig. 6.4

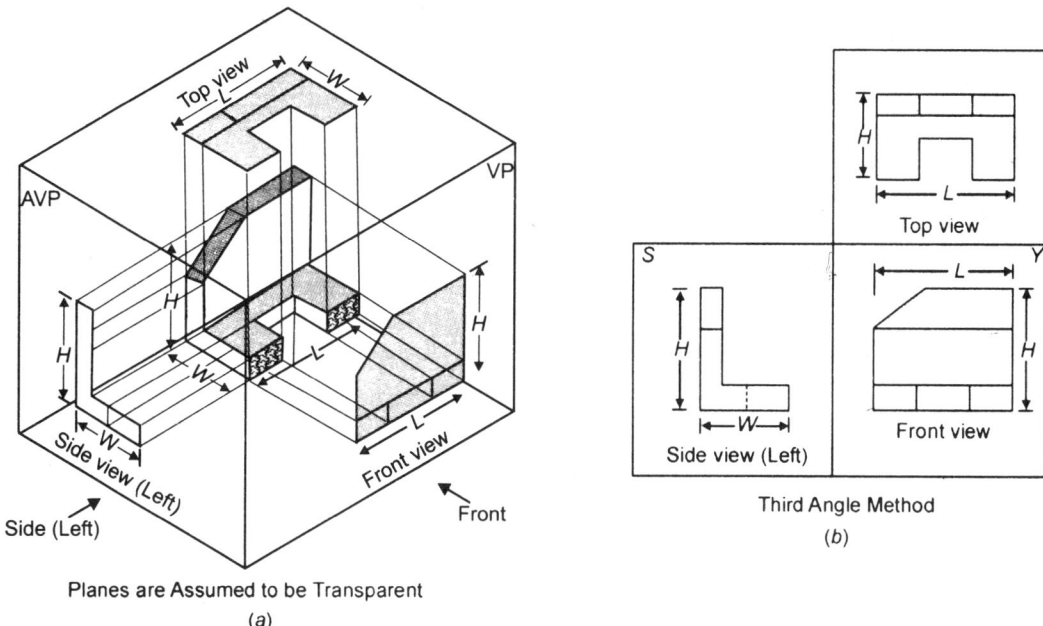

Planes are Assumed to be Transparent

(a)

Third Angle Method

(b)

Fig. 6.5

Table: Differences between first-angle projection method and third-angle projection method.

S. No.	First-angle projection method	Third-angle projection method
1.	The object is kept in the first quadrant.	The object is assumed to be kept in the third quadrant.
2.	The object lies between the observer and the plane of projection.	The plane of projection lies between the observer and the object.
3.	The plane of projection is assumed to be *non-transparent*.	To plane of projection is assumed to be transparent.
4.	In this method, when the views are drawn in their relative positions, the plan (top view) comes below the elevation, the view of the object as observed from the left-side is drawn to the right of elevation.	In this method, when the views are drawn in their relative positions, the plan (top view), comes above the elevation, left hand side view is drawn to the left hand side of the elevation.
5.	This method of projection is now recommended by the "Bureau of Indian Standards" from 1991.	This method of projection is used in USA and also in other countries.
6.	It is represented by the symbol	It is represented by the symbol

Conversion of Pictorial View into Orthographic Views

Pictorial view is a three-dimensional view of an object. It does not show the true shape of its surfaces. Hidden parts and constructional details are not clearly shown. Therefore such parts are to be imagined.

In orthographic projections, only two dimensions are seen in the front view, top view and side view. The width (W) will not be seen in the front view, as the observer looks at the object parallel to the width of the object. For top view he looks parallel to the height of the object, hence height (H) will not be seen in the top view. As he looks parallel to the length of the object for side view, the length (L) will not be seen in that view.

The following points are to be remembered in connection with the pictorial view.
- The hidden part of a symmetrical object is to be treated similar to the visible part.
- The holes, grooves, etc. are assumed to be drilled or cut right through, unless otherwise specified.
- When the radii for small curves of fillets are not specified, they are to be assumed.

The following points are to be considered while converting the pictorial view into orthographic views.
- The direction of the front view is the front direction and it is generally indicated by an arrow. The direction of side view (left or right) is decided from the front direction.
- The edges of the object parallel to the direction of the observer will be seen as points.
- The surfaces parallel to the direction of the observer will be seen as lines.
- The surface at right angles to the direction of the observer will be represented by the true shape of the surface. The sloping surface perpendicular to the direction of vision will be represented by a sloping line, whereas the curved surface will be shown by a curved line.
- The invisible edges of the object are to be represented by dotted lines.
- Having decided the direction of side view (either left or right), fix up the relative positions of the front view, top view and side view according to the method of projection used. While using third angle of projection, top view must be located exactly above the front view and the side view from left must be located to the left side of the front view as shown in Fig. 6.5 (*a* and *b*).
- Study the shape and dimensions of the object and determine the overall dimensions for each view. Take a convenient scale for drawing so as to accommodate the views in the drawing sheet.
- Using H pencil and with light hand, layout the rectangles for the views. Sufficient space must be kept between them (i.e. about 30 to 40 mm maximum).
- Draw the centre lines in all the views for details.

- First start drawing the view in which the circular parts of the object are seen as circles or part of it. It becomes simpler to project the points of the circle in other views.
- Draw straight lines.
- Locate intersections and small curves and complete the views.
- Rub out all unnecessary lines.
- Fair the views with 2H or 3H pencil. The outline should be uniformly thick and dark.
- Draw section lines in the sectional view, if any.
- Dimension the views.
- Name the view.
- Print the title and scale.

ISOMETRIC PROJECTION

In isometric projection, the three edges of a solid right angle of an object are shown by means of three line drawn from a point and parallel to the three isometric axes which meet at a point and make an angle of 120° with each other. The vertical edge of the solid right angle is shown by a vertical line while the two horizontal edges are shown by two lines inclined at 30° to the horizontal. While rectangles are drawn as parallelograms having sides parallel to two of the three axes and having included angles of 60° and 120°. Thus, in an isometric view a right angle is shown by a 60° or 120° angles and circles are shown as ellipses. In isometric projections, the direction of viewing is such that three axes of space (length, width and height) appears foreshortened and hence only one scale is used.

Problem

Pictorial view is given in Fig. 6.6. Draw to full size scale, the following views by Third Angle Method of Projection:

1. Front view looking in the direction *X*,
2. Top view and
3. Side view looking from right.

Procedure to draw an isometric view of a solid

- Assume that front view, top view and side view are rectangles *ABED*, *DEGM* and *CADM* respectively.
- Draw a base line.
- Draw a line *AB* at 30° to base line on one side and line *AC* at 30° on the other side and *AD* vertical to base line, to natural scale.
- Complete the box (cuboid).
- In the longer sides of the top surface of this box, locate points *H*, *K*, *L*, *N* at given distances from ends of the sides.
- Draw vertical lines through *H* and *N* (parallel to *AD*) and mark *Q* and *R* at distances 20 mm from *H* and *N* respectively.

- Join *QR*, this line will be parallel to *AB*.
- Draw lines parallel to *HK* from points *Q* and *R* (the line through *R* will not be seen).
- Draw vertical lines from *K* and *L* to obtain intersection points at the back of *Q* and *R* (the line through *L* will not be seen).

The completed isometric view is shown in the Fig. 6.6(*b*).

Some selected problems are completely solved, which the students will find useful for understanding isometric projections. The students should study them critically and practice.

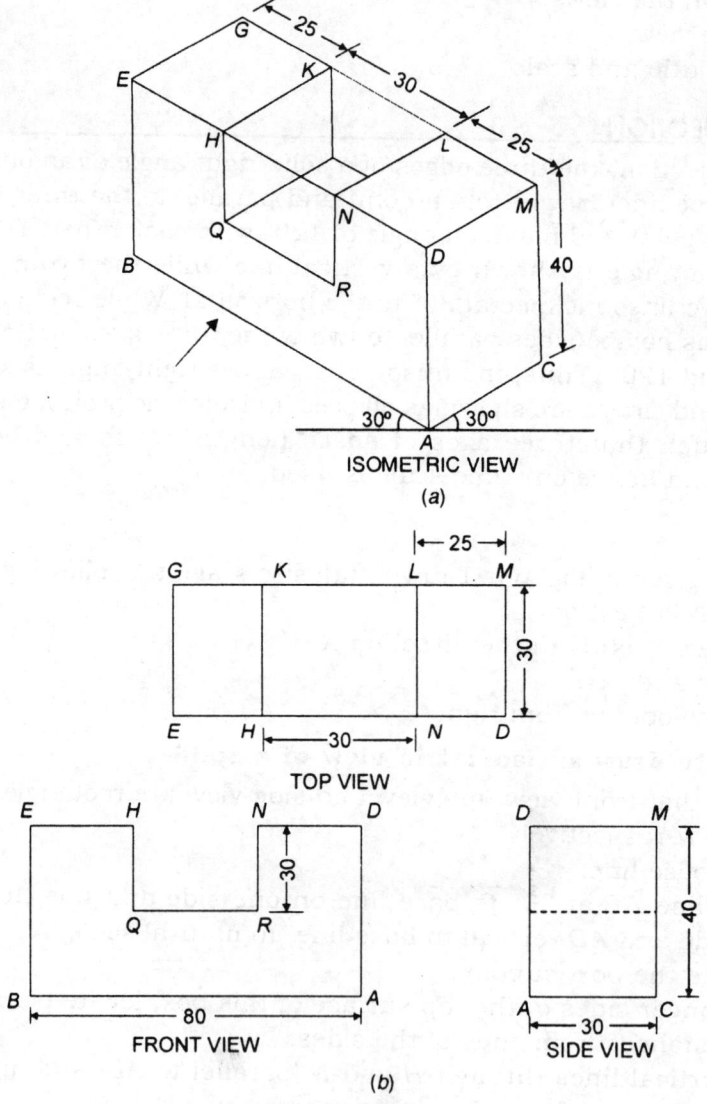

Fig. 6.6

Problems

Figure shows a pictorial view of an object. Using full size scale, draw the following views by Third Angle Method of projection:

1. Front view looking in the direction of arrow *X*,
2. Top view and
3. Side view looking from right.

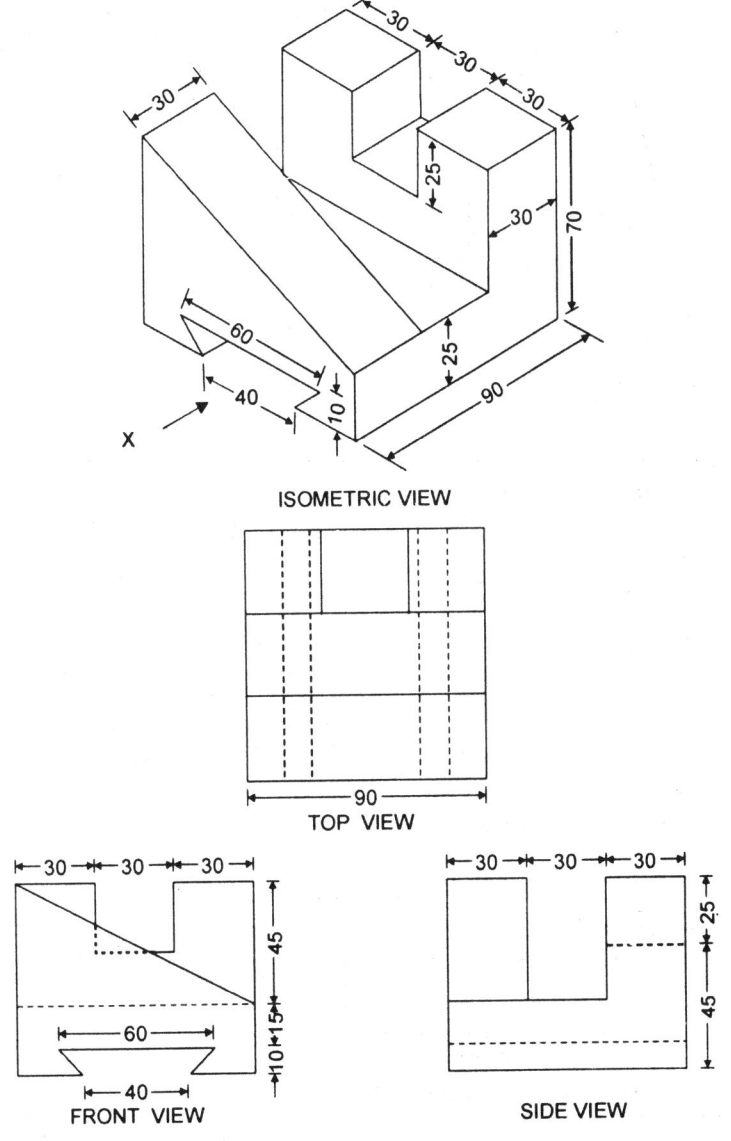

ISOMETRIC VIEW

TOP VIEW

FRONT VIEW

SIDE VIEW

1. Draw isometric view, front view, top view and side view by first angle method of projection.

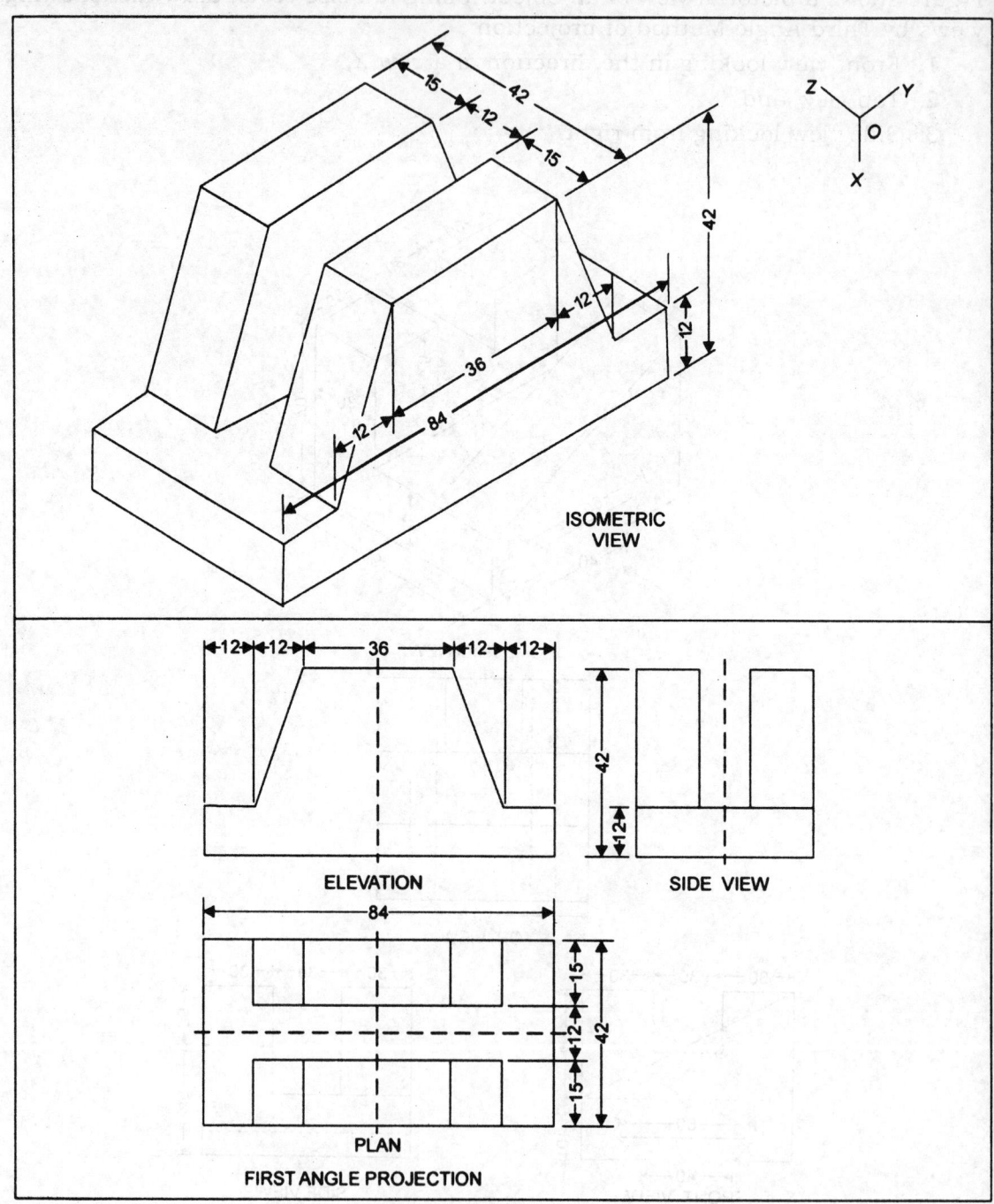

2. Draw isometric view, front view, top view and side view by third angle method of projection.

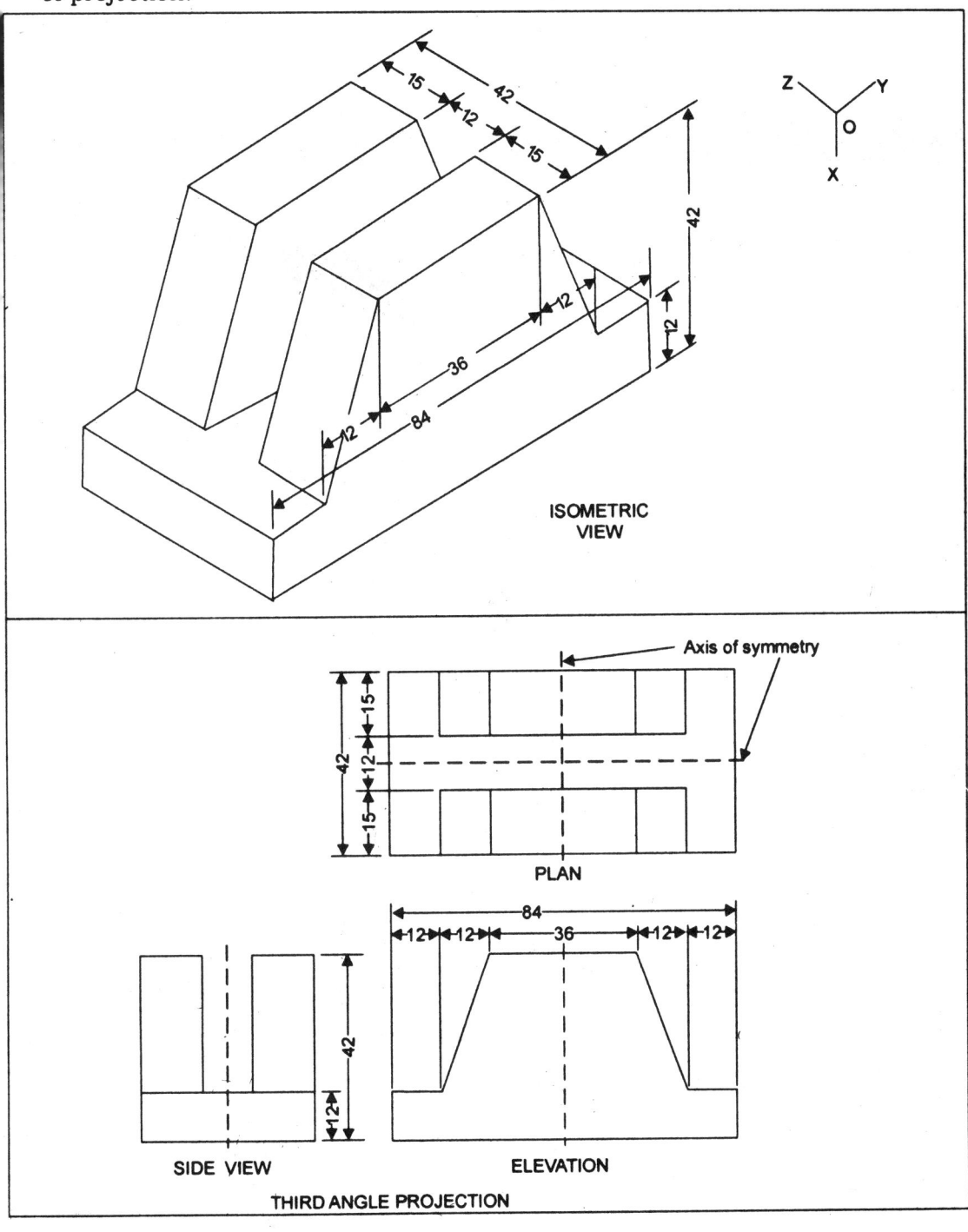

ISOMETRIC
VIEW

Axis of symmetry

PLAN

SIDE VIEW

ELEVATION

THIRD ANGLE PROJECTION

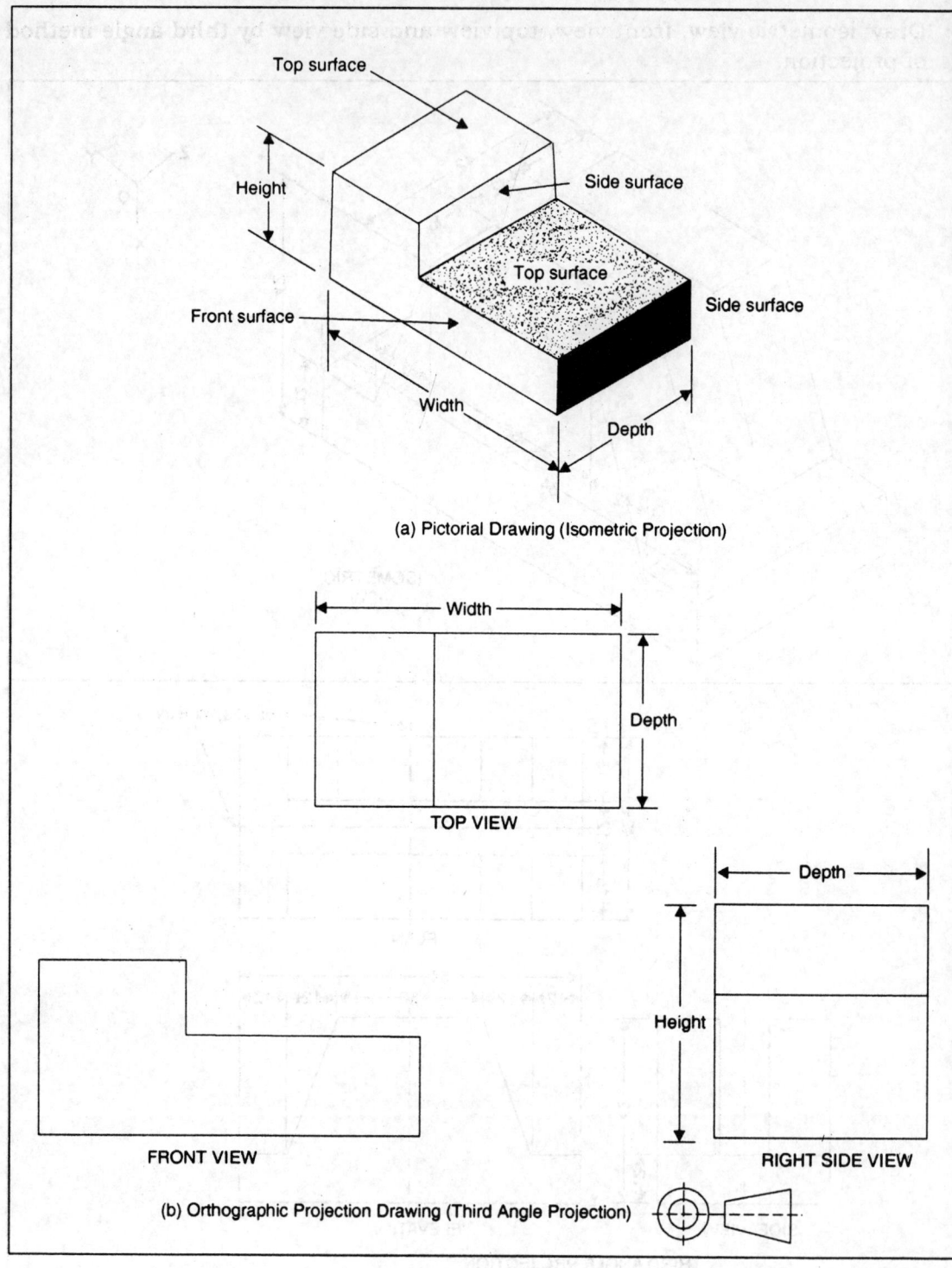

Top surface

Side surface

Height

Top surface

Side surface

Front surface

Width

Depth

(a) Pictorial Drawing (Isometric Projection)

Width

Depth

TOP VIEW

Depth

Height

FRONT VIEW

RIGHT SIDE VIEW

(b) Orthographic Projection Drawing (Third Angle Projection)

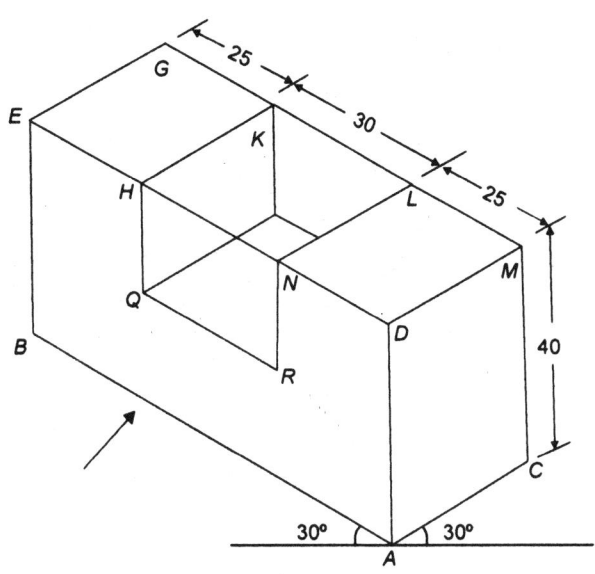

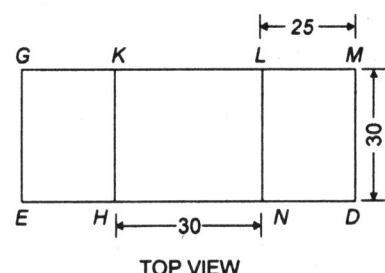

TOP VIEW

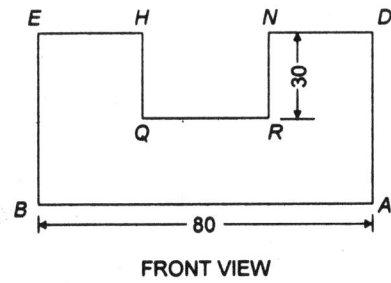

FRONT VIEW

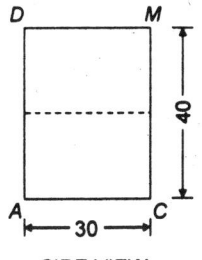

SIDE VIEW

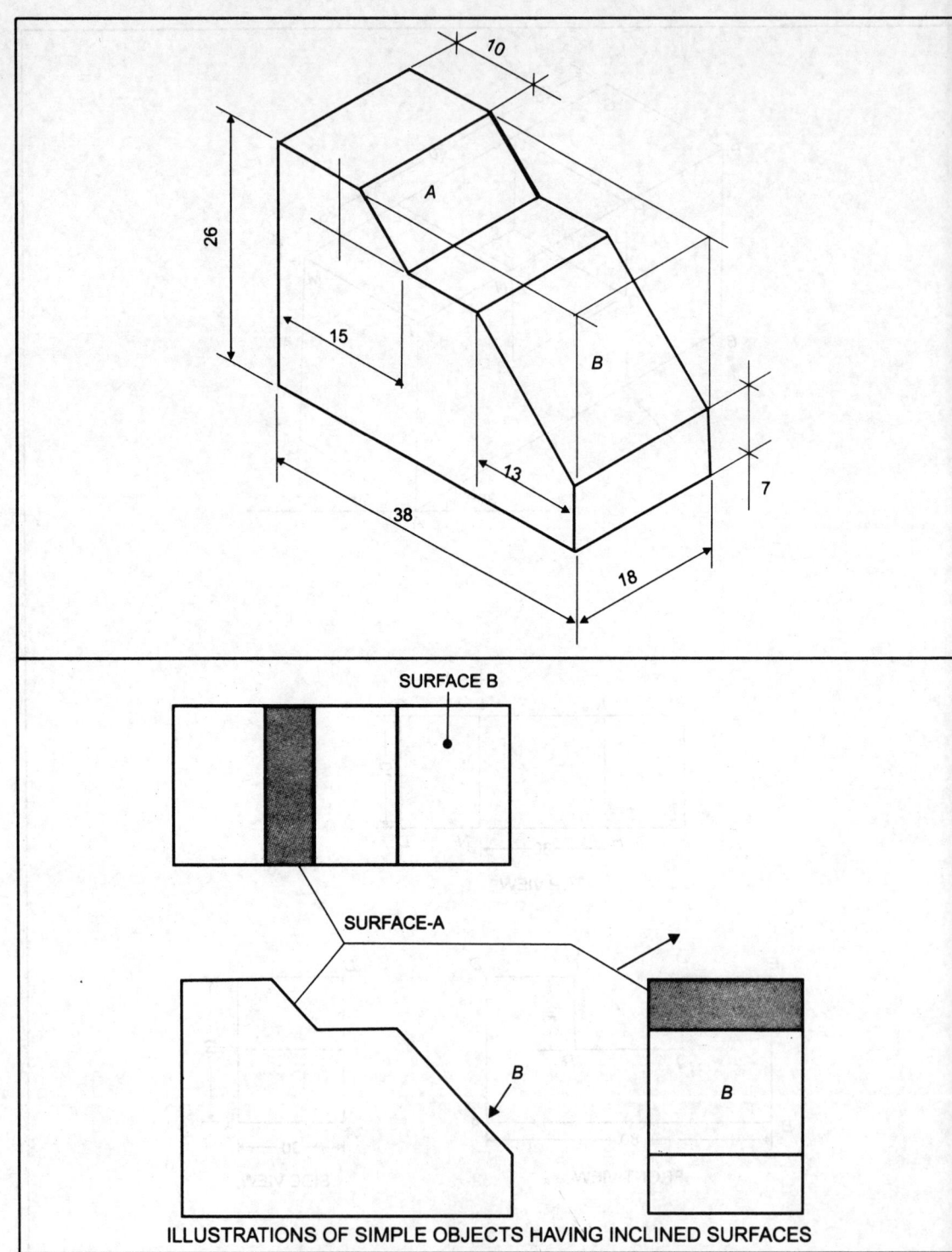

SURFACE B

SURFACE-A

ILLUSTRATIONS OF SIMPLE OBJECTS HAVING INCLINED SURFACES

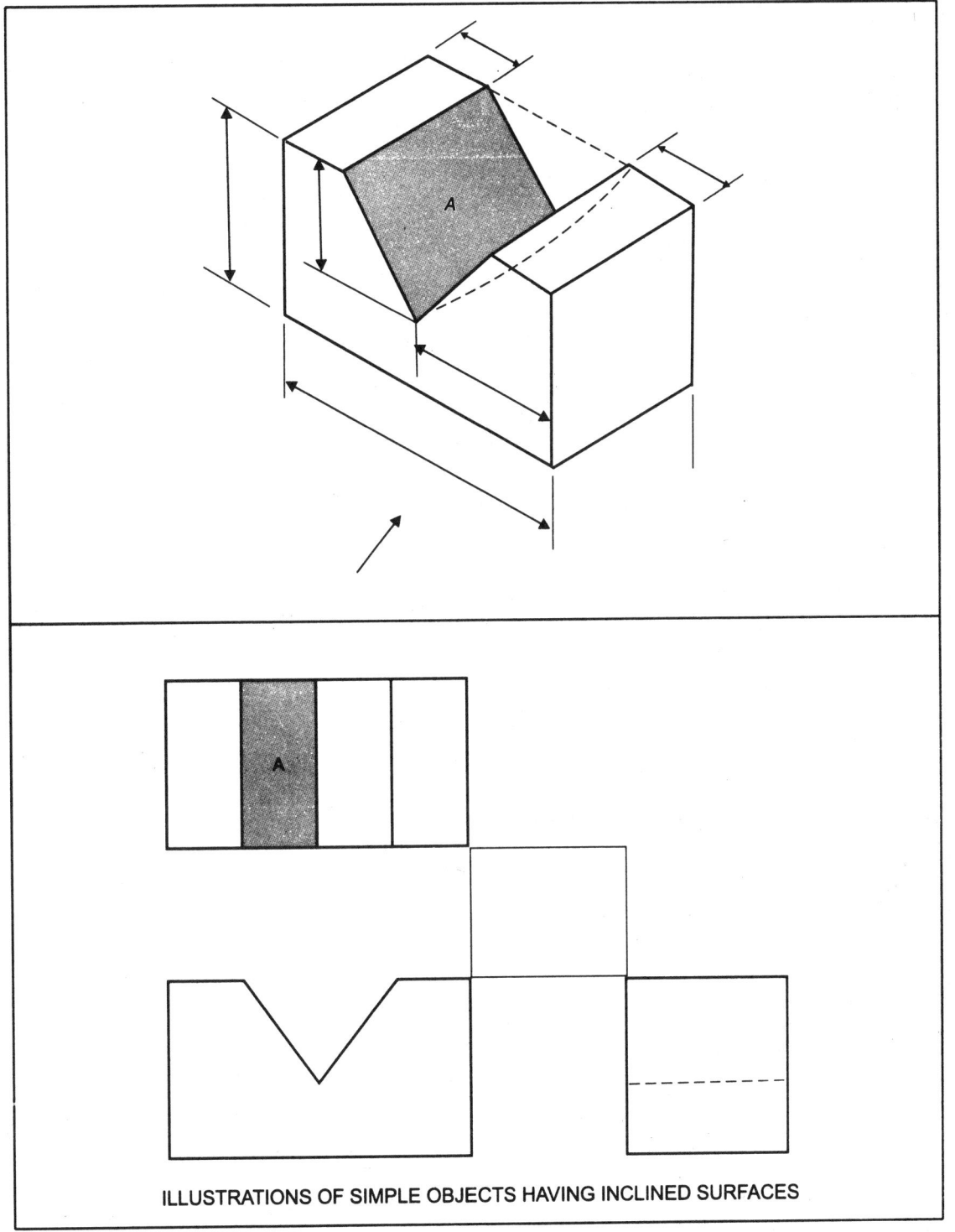

ILLUSTRATIONS OF SIMPLE OBJECTS HAVING INCLINED SURFACES

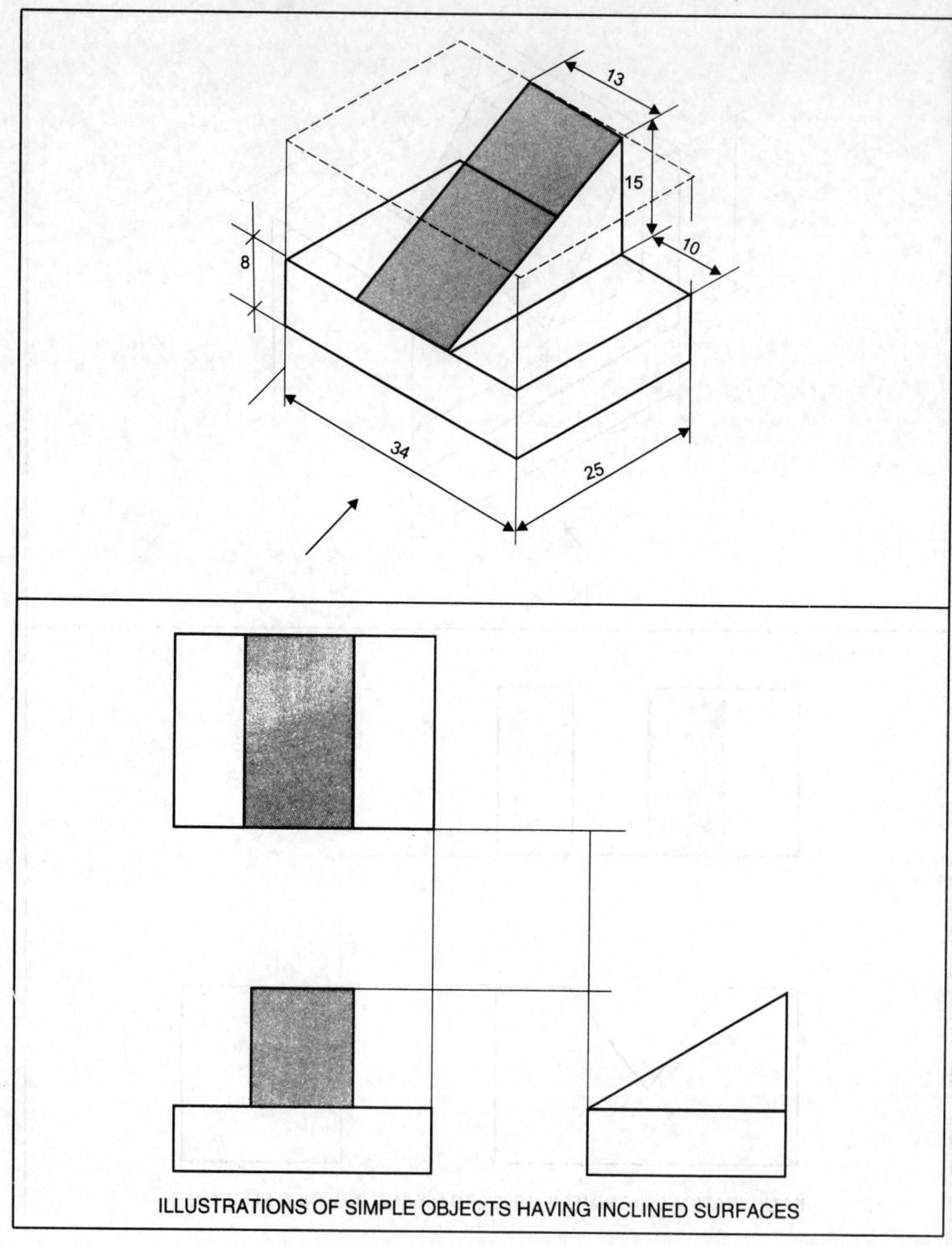

ILLUSTRATIONS OF SIMPLE OBJECTS HAVING INCLINED SURFACES

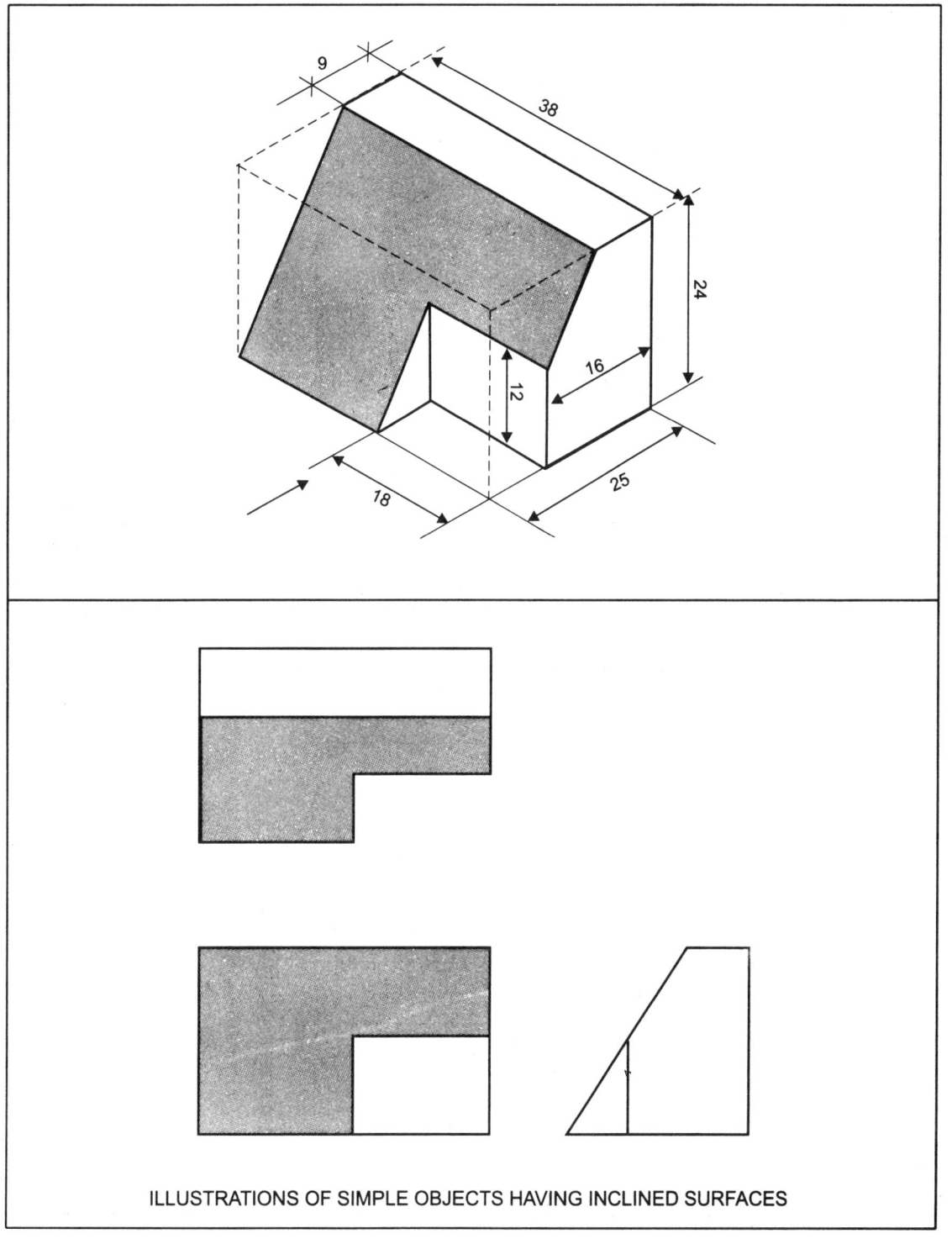

ILLUSTRATIONS OF SIMPLE OBJECTS HAVING INCLINED SURFACES

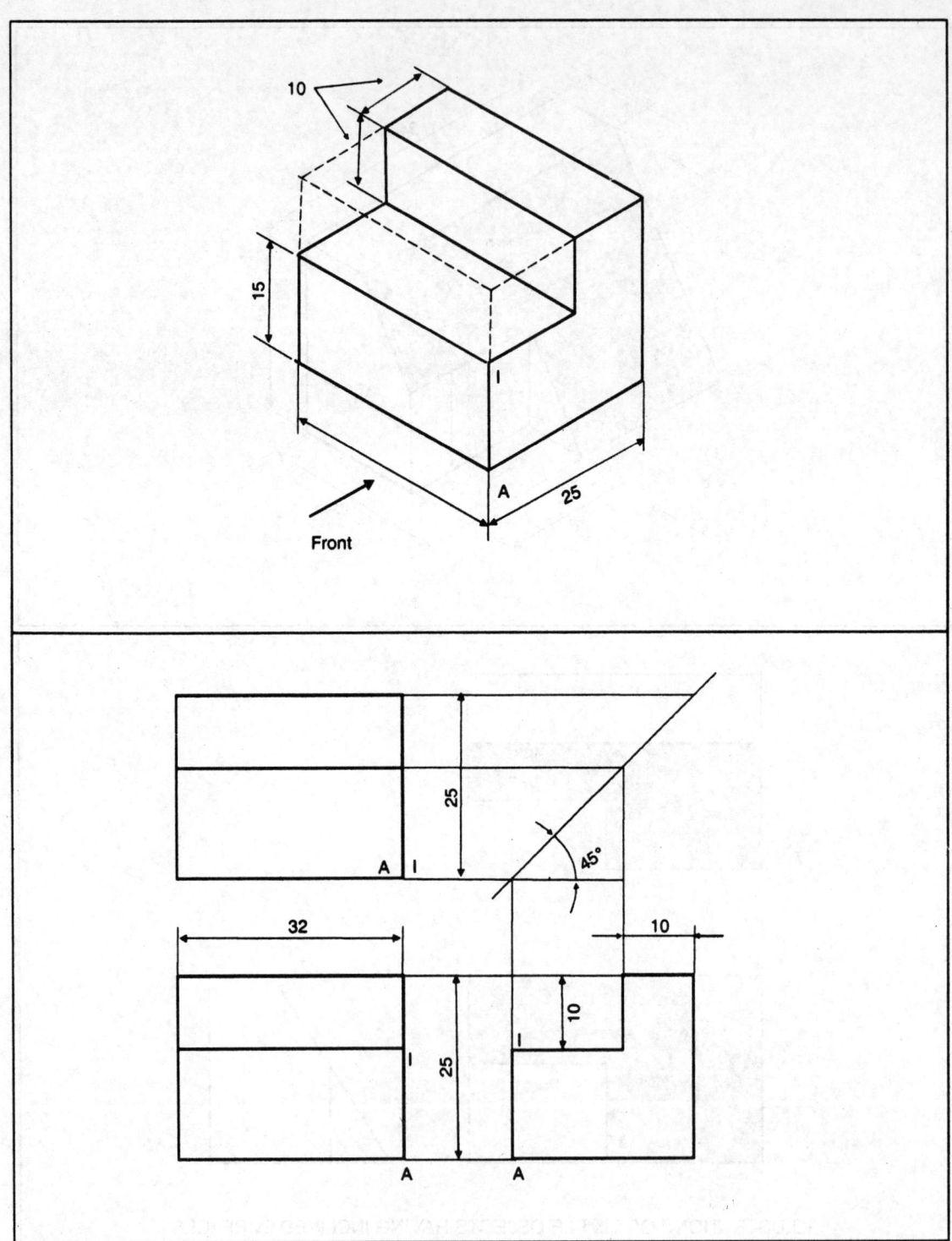

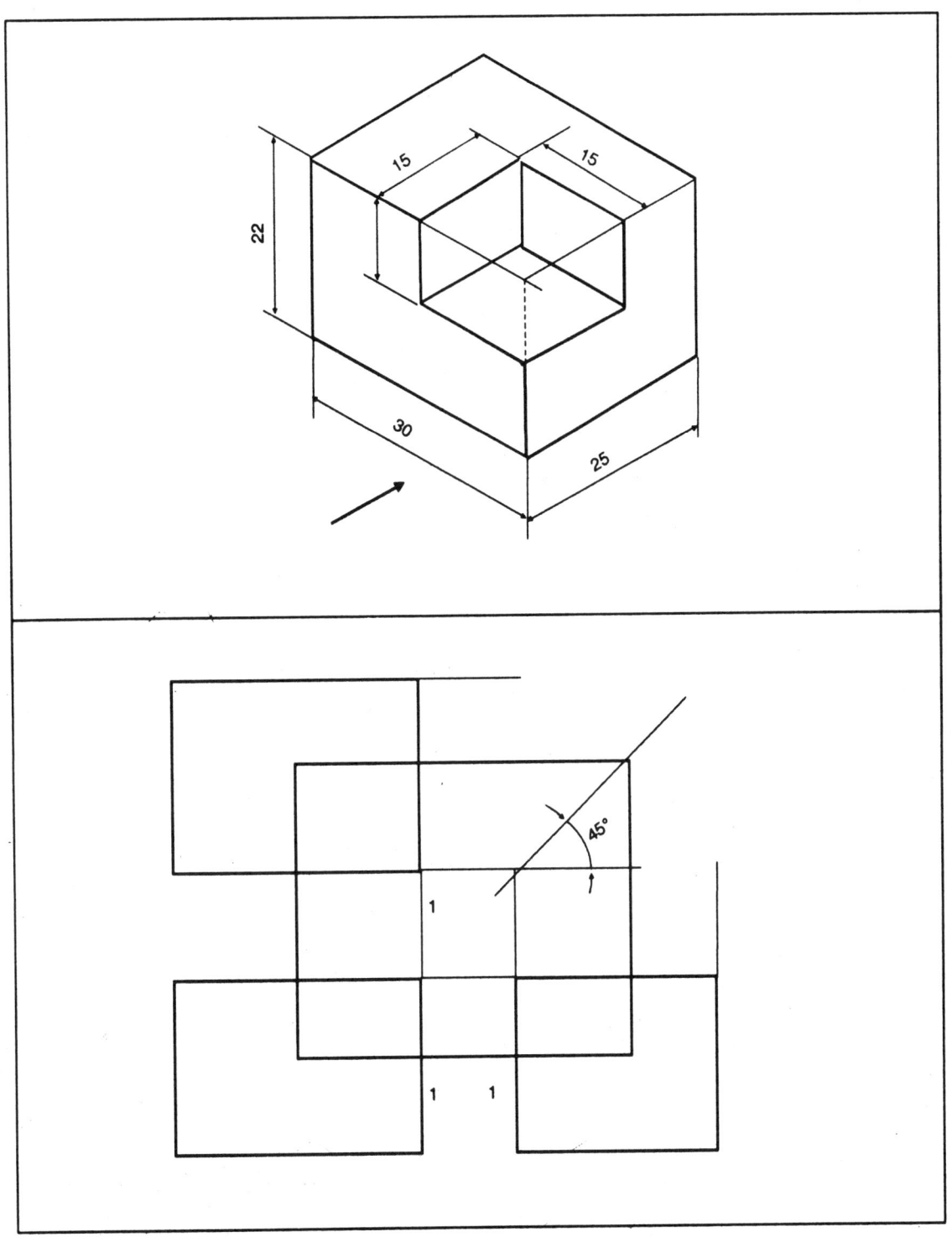

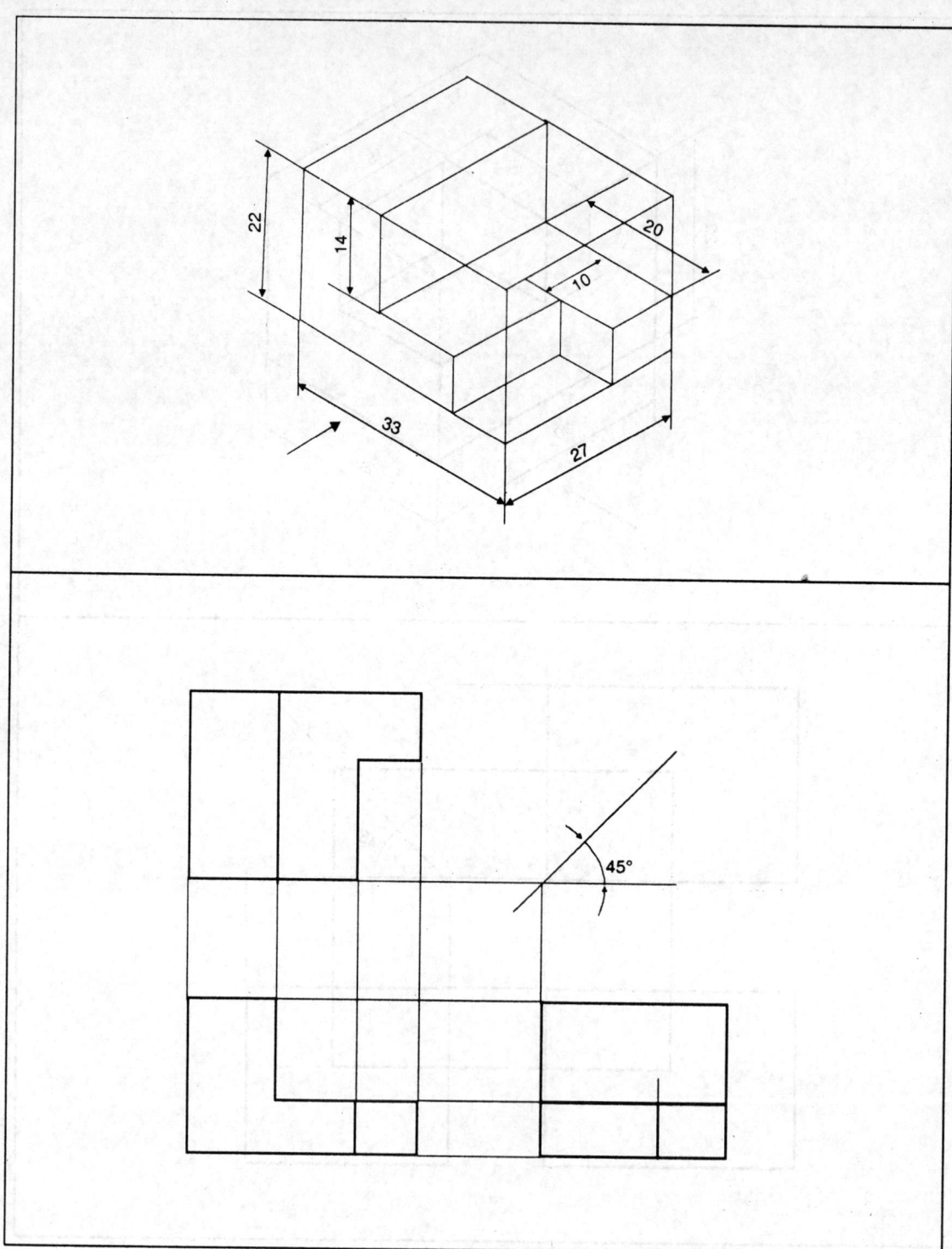

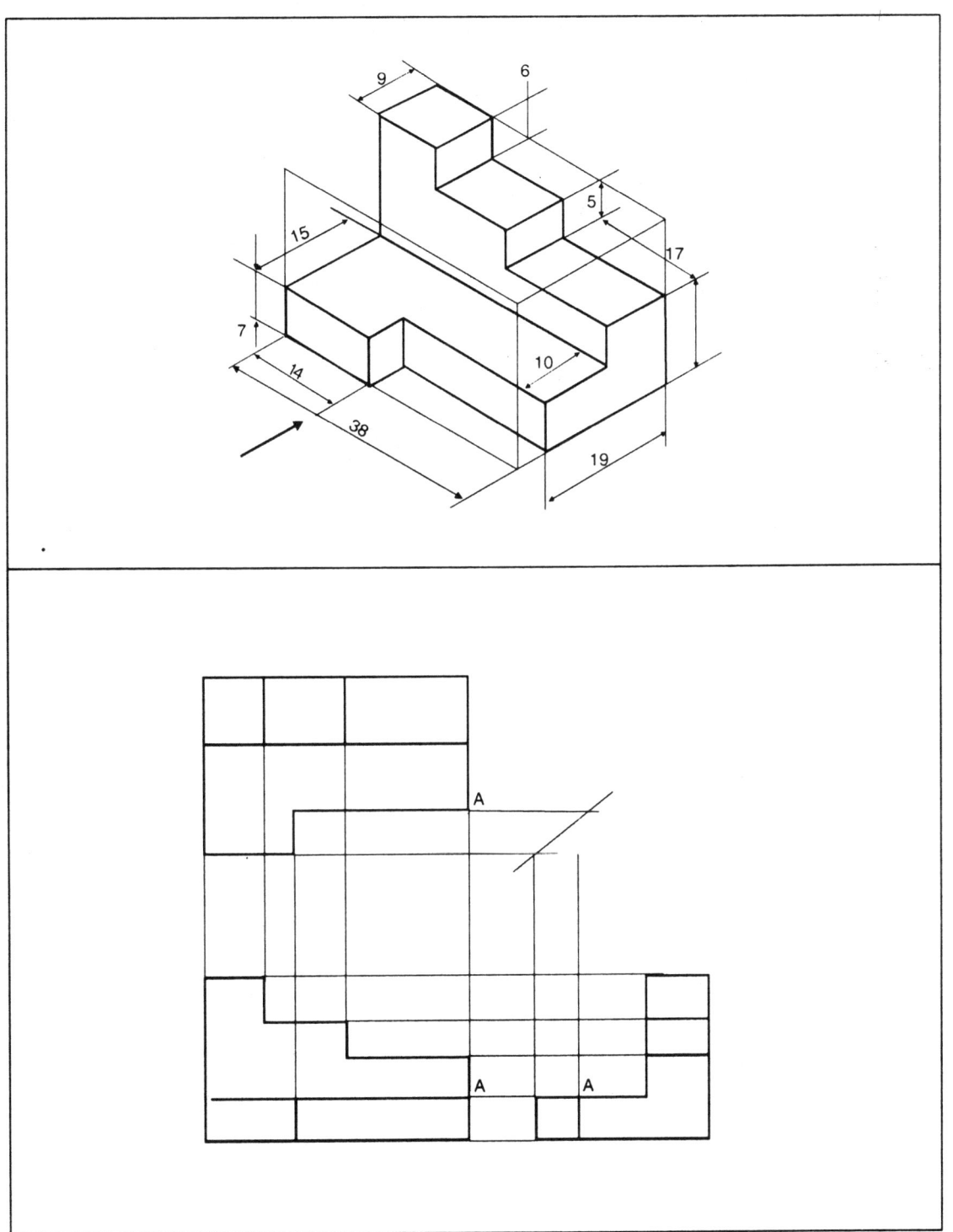

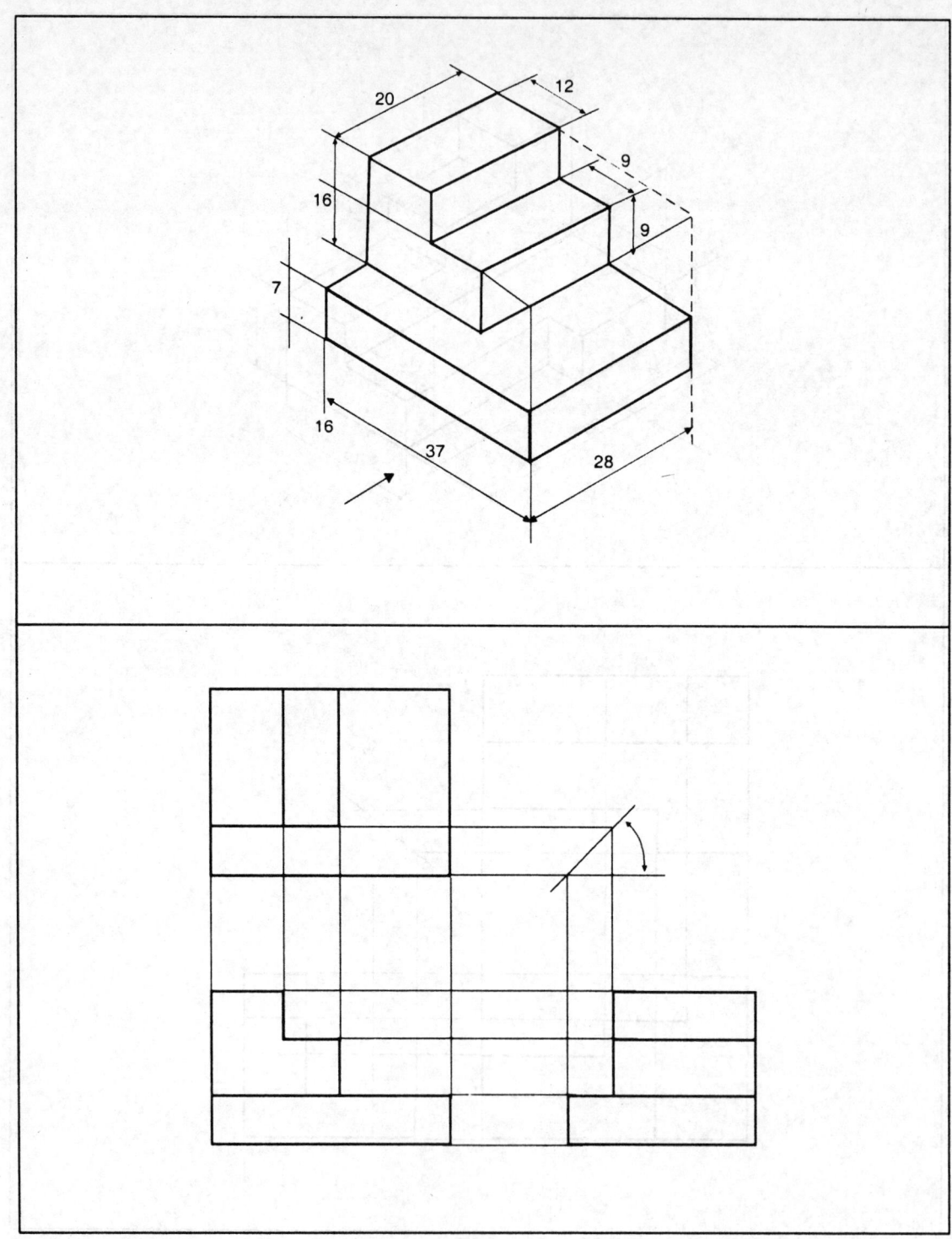

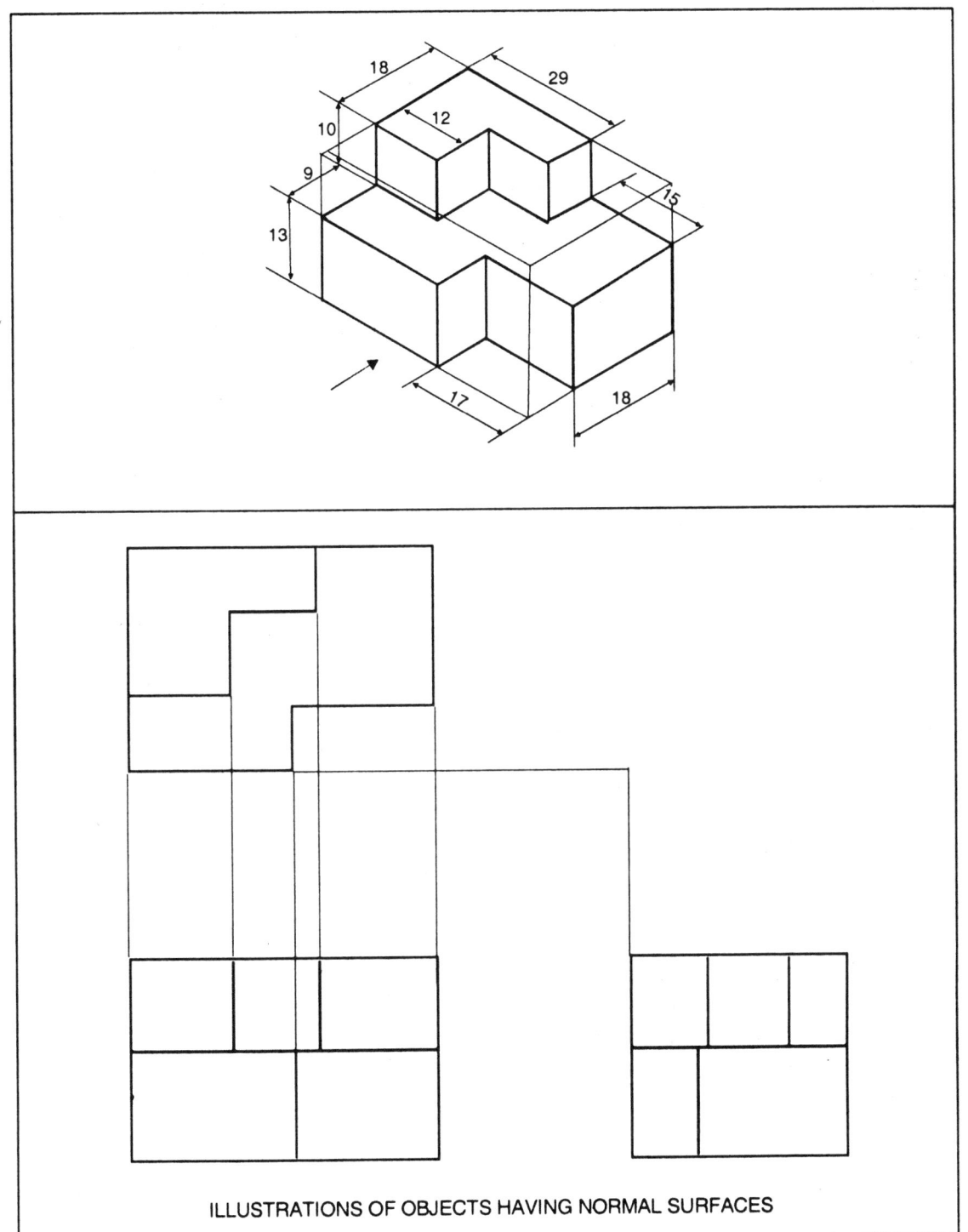

ILLUSTRATIONS OF OBJECTS HAVING NORMAL SURFACES

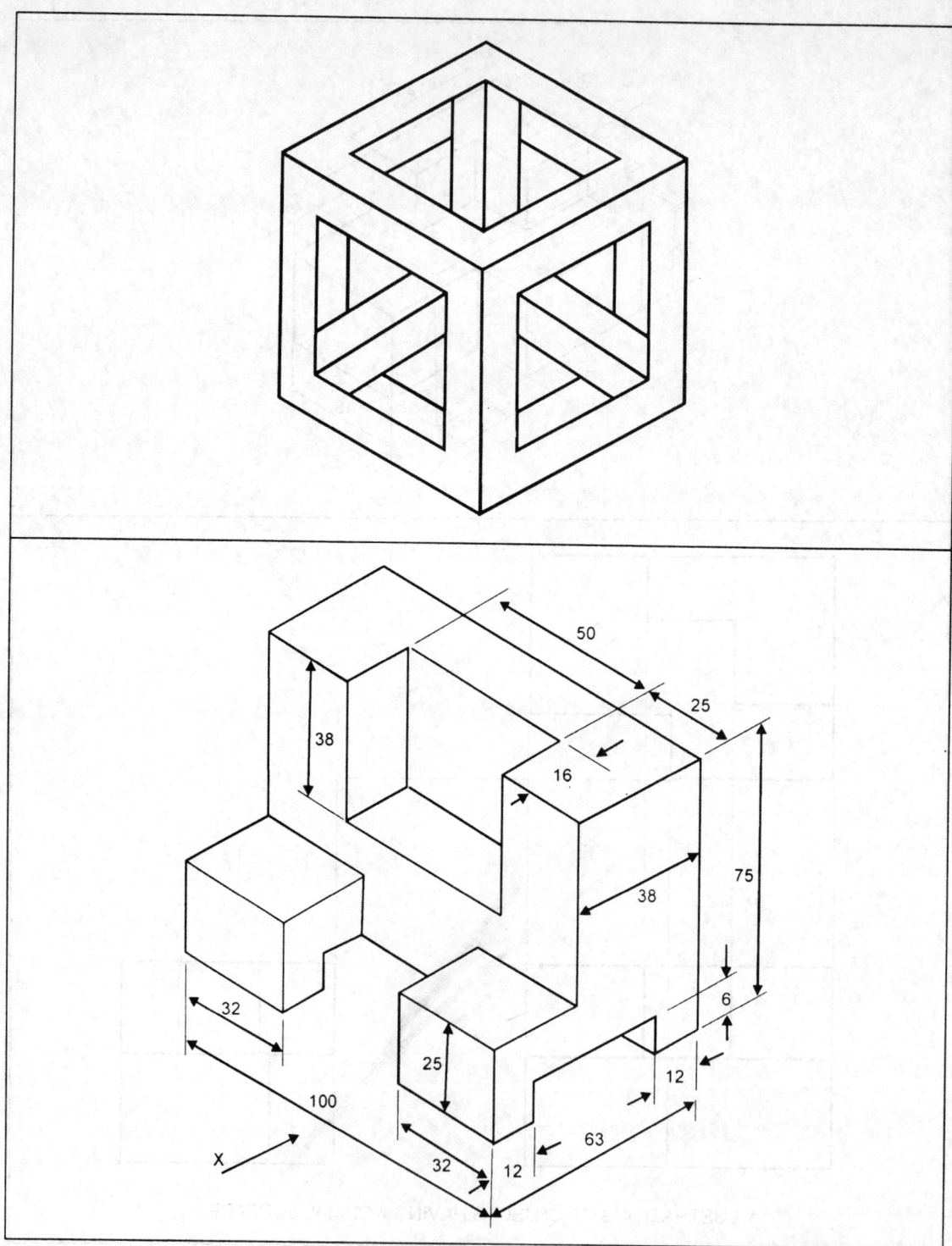

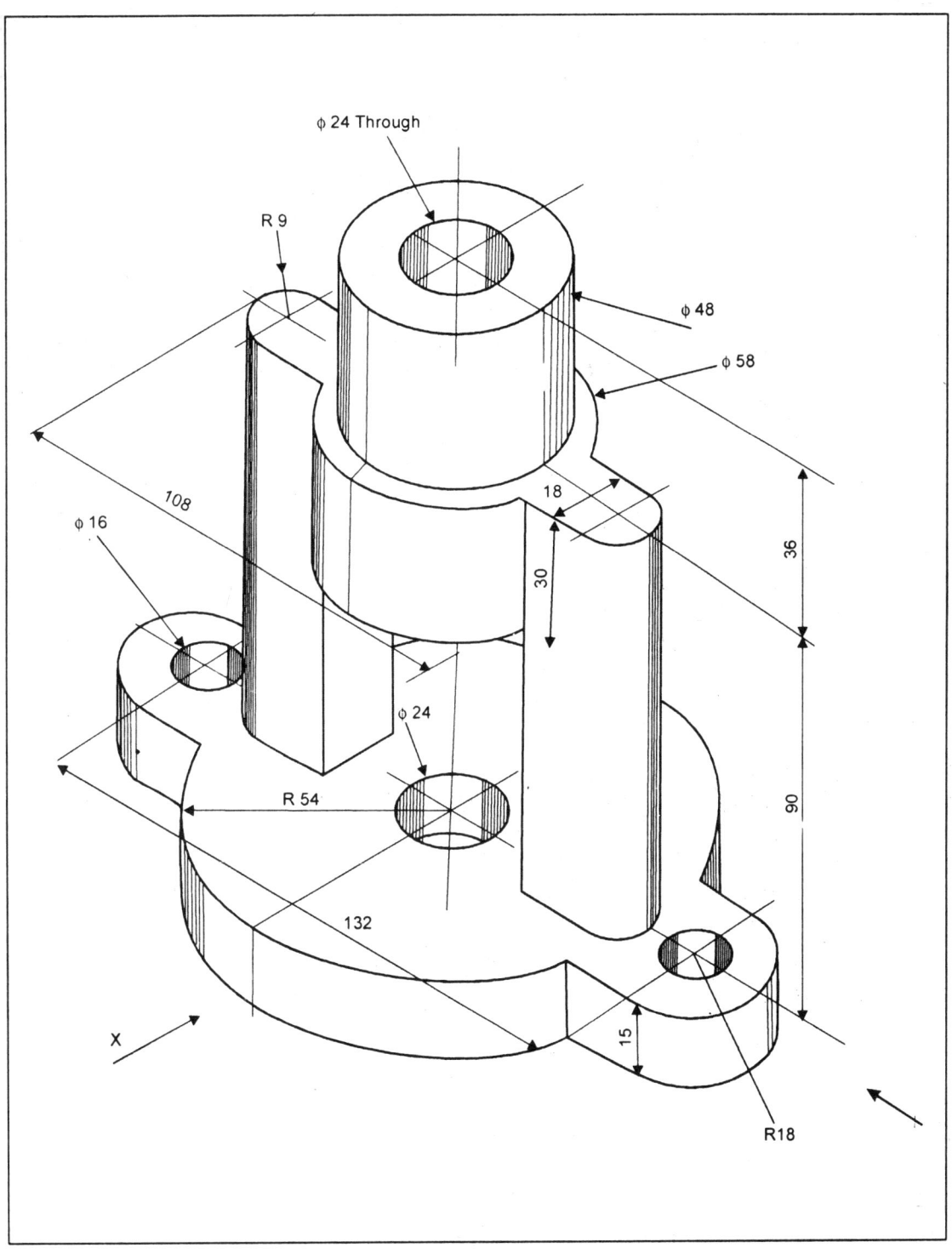

Oil Hole 3 Dia, C′ sunk 3 at 45°
40 R
22
45
20
30
45
140
60
30

16
8
10
12
8
20
20
16
16
20
8
32
56
X

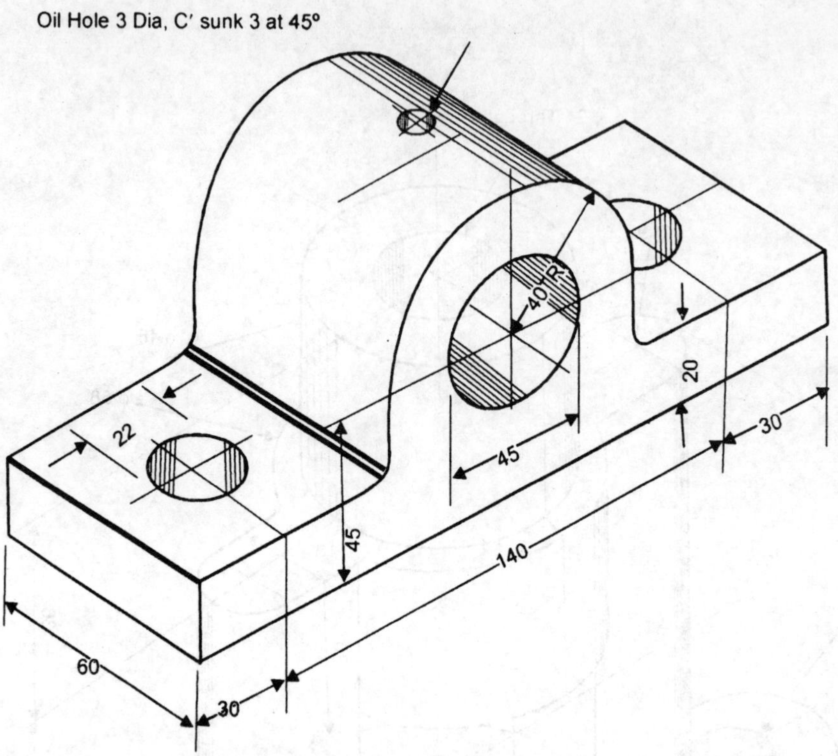

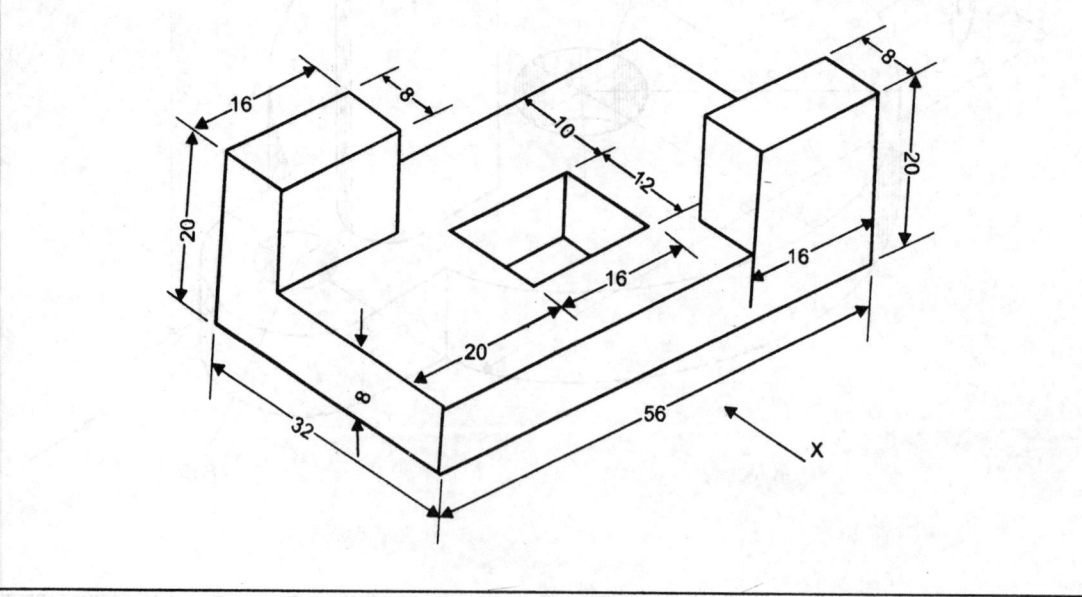

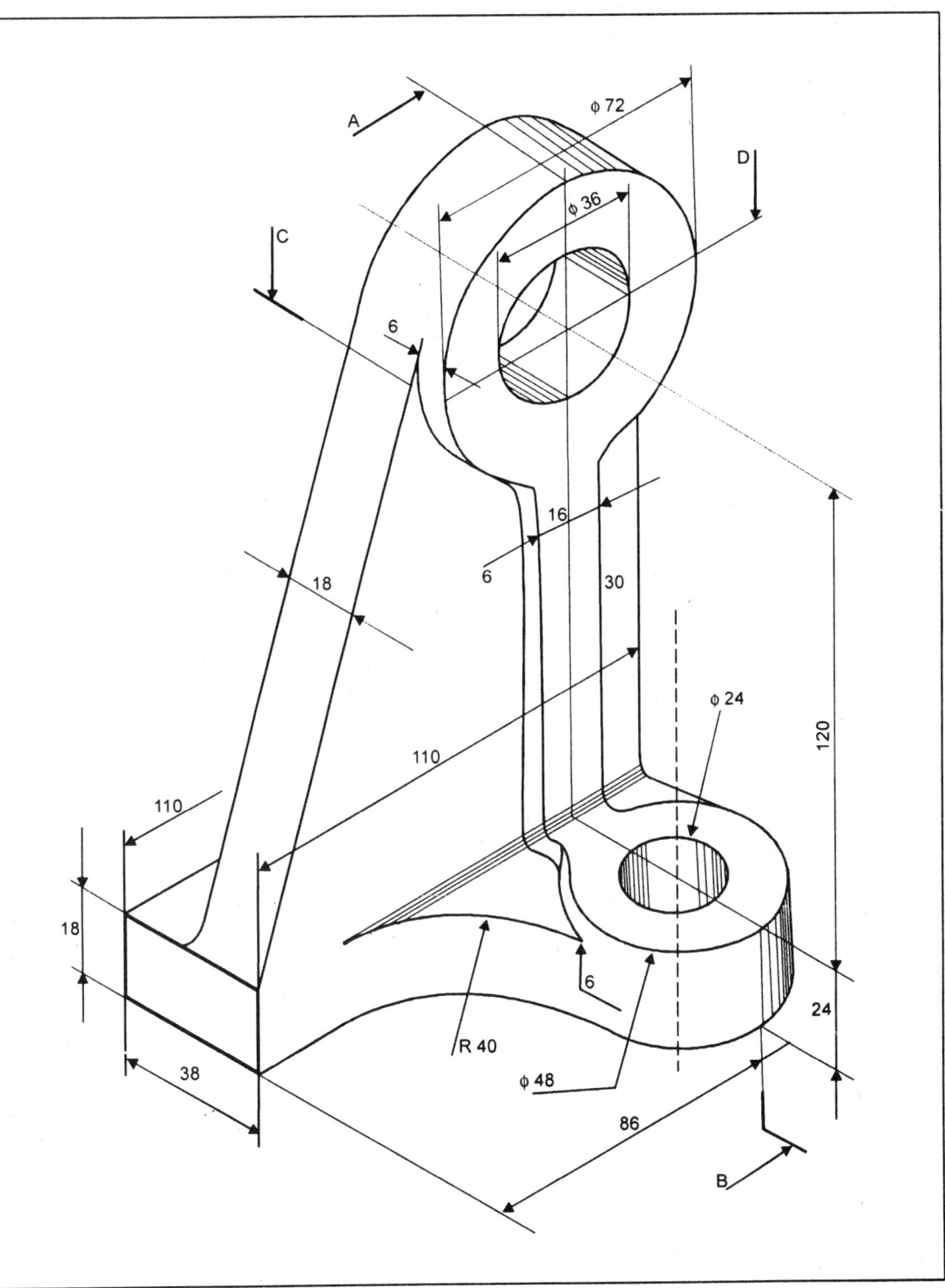

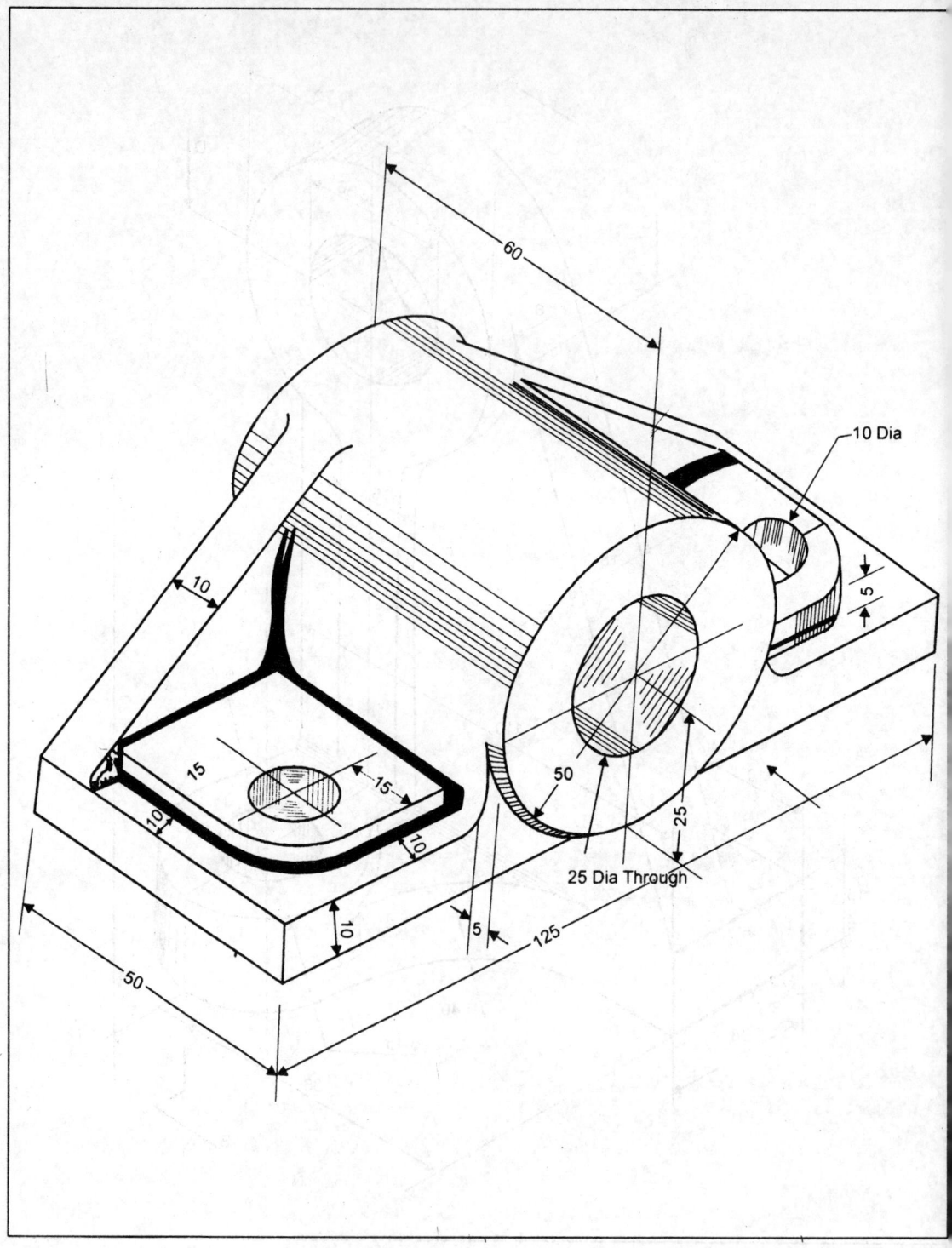

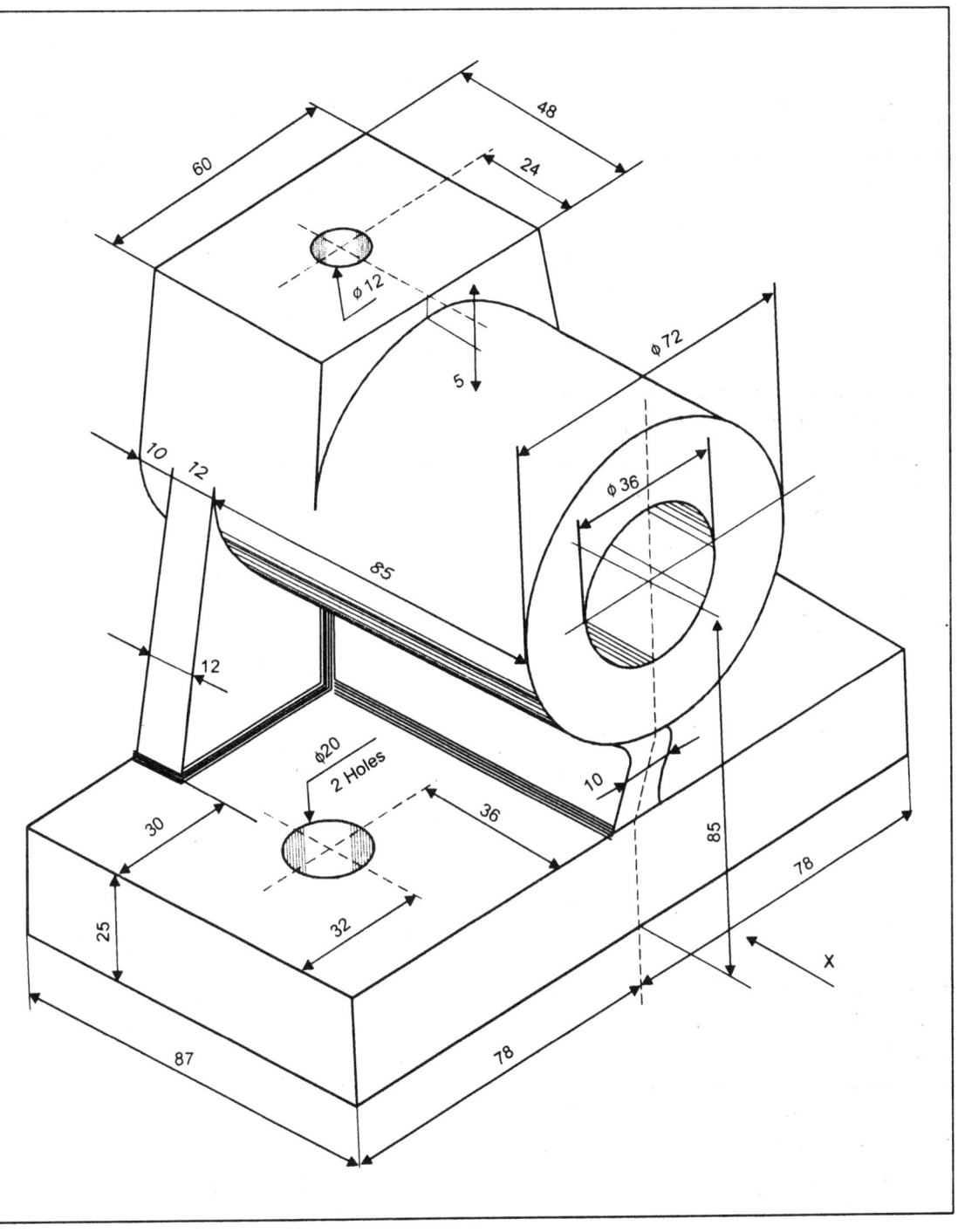

7

Nuts and Bolts

Freehand sketching and preparation of drawings of nuts and bolts and simple blueprint reading

Bolts and nuts, studs and nuts are widely used for temporary fastening of two or more parts together. Figure 7.1 shows nut and bolt.

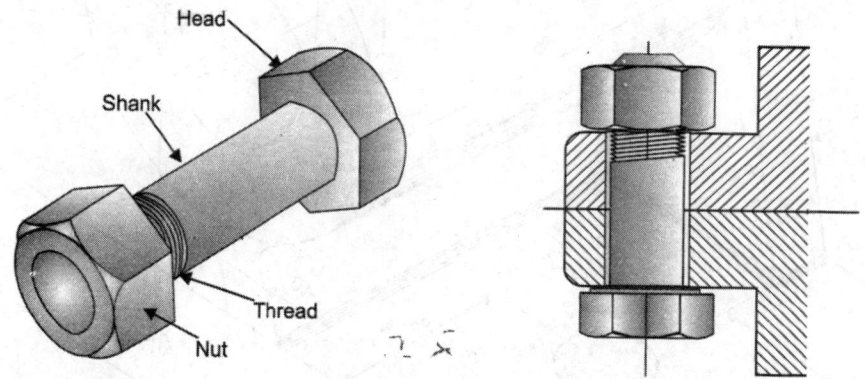

Fig. 7.1: *Nut and bolt*

NUTS

Nuts are generally in the form of hexagonal or square prisms. Besides these, cylindrical and other forms are also used. In the hexagonal nut, the upper corners of this nut is rounded-off or chamfered. The chamfering is generally conical. The angle of chamfer is 30° or 45° with the base of the nut. Due to chamfering, an arc is formed on each vertical face and a circle is formed on the top surface of the nut.

The dimensions of the hexagonal nut cannot be expressed exactly in terms of the nominal diameter of the bolt. For calculation of standard proportions of nuts and bolts, the following calculation may be adopted:

If D = the nominal diameter of the bolt

Thickness of the nut T = D

Width across flats, W = $1.5D + 3$ mm

Angle of chamfer = 30°

Radius of chamfer arc, R = $1.4D$ approx.

Very often and especially when a nut is shown in one view only, the following rough rule dimensions of chamfer arc, R = $1.5D$ approx.

Thickness of the nut T = D

Width across diagonally opposite corners = 2

Angle of chamfer = 30°

Radius of chamfer arc, R = $1.4D$ approx.

TYPES OF NUTS

Dome Nut

It is the type of a hexagonal nut, closed at one and with a spherical dome at the top, which protects the end of the bolt from being corroded.

Cap Nut

This is also a form of a hexagonal nut, closed at one end with a cylindrical cap at the top, which prevents leakage through the threads.

Capstan Nut

It is a form of a cylindrical nut with circular holes on the curved surface, which are used for turning it with a tommy bar.

Wing Nut

It is a form of a conical nut with two wings which can be easily operated by the thumb and finger for frequent adjustment.

Cup Head Bolt

It is in the form of a cup with a snug forged on the shank which enables it to fit into a similar recess in the hole to prevent the bolt from rotating.

Countersunk Head Bolt

This type of bolt is used in cases where the heed of a bolt should not project above the surface of the body. It may be provided with a snug or square neck to prevent the rotation of the bolt.

Hook Bolt

This type of bolt has its head protected to one side of its shank. It grips the end of one part and passes through a hole in the other part. Its square neck prevent the rotation of the bolt.

Eye Bolt

It has a circular ring for its head, hence, its rotation can be prevented by passing or holding a rod through it.

Problem

To draw a top view and project three views of a given nut for a bolt of diameter D.

Solution

Nuts and Bolts

Approximate Properties for Ordinary Nut

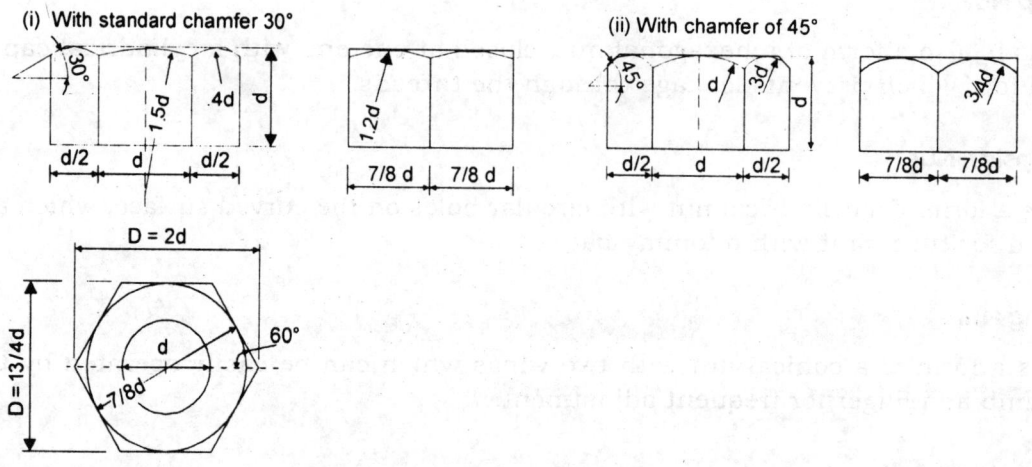

Fig. 7.2

Forms of bolts

(*i*) Assume rough-rule dimensions.

Hexagonal-headed bolt : *This is the most common form* of a bolt. The hexagonal head is chamfered at its upper end. To prevent rotation of the bolt while screwing the nut on or off it, the bolt-head is held by another spanner.

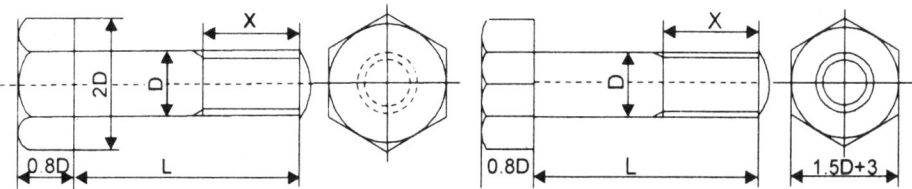

***Fig. 7.3:** Hexagonal-headed bolt*

The dimensions of the bolt-head are the same as those of the hexagonal nut, except for the thickness. For elementary work, the thickness is taken as 0.8*D* to *D* and figures show two views each of a hexagonal-headed bolt drawn according to *rough-rule dimensions and approximately standard dimensions respectively. Note that the length of the face of the bolt-head is equal to D in figure, while it is less than D in figure.*

Problem

To draw three views of a hexagonal-headed bolt, 24 mm diameter and 100 mm long, with a hexagonal nut and a washer.

(*i*) Assume rough-rule dimensions.

(*ii*) Determine the dimensions of the nut and the washer as shown below.

Dimensions for the nut:	Dimensions for washer:
Thickness of the nut = 24 mm	Diameter of the washer = 52 mm
Distance across diagonally:	Thickness = 3 mm
Opposite corners = 48 mm	Diameter of the hole = 24.5 mm
Angle of chamfer = 30°	
Radius of chamfer arc, *R* = 36 mm.	

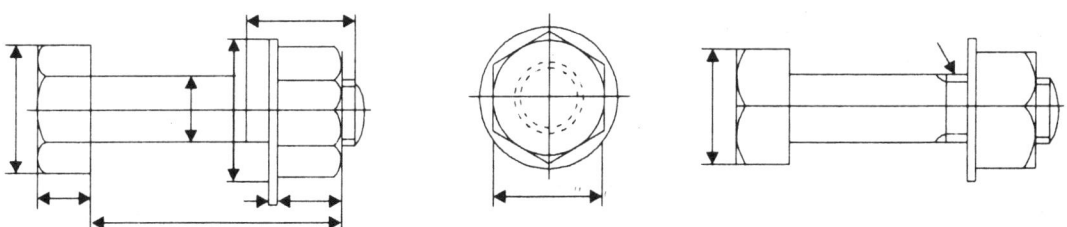

***Fig. 7.4:** Hexagonal-headed bolt with hexagonal nut and washer*

Step 1: Draw the horizontal centre line and around it construct a rectangle *100 mm × 24 mm for the shank.*

Step 2: Add the view of the bolt-head and the nut showing three faces. *The distance between the outer edges will be 48 mm.*

Step 3: Draw the chamfer arcs, etc.

Step 4: *Draw the rectangle for the washer, 52 mm × 3 mm, attached to* the nut.

Step 5: The end of the bolt is usually rounded. It is drawn by a radius equal to the diameter of the bolt.

Step 6: Project the side view and the top view. The width *W* across the flats will be equal to $\sqrt{3}$ × 24 mm.

(*iii*) When drawing the views according to approximately standard dimensions, beginning must be made with the hexagon in the side view and the other views must then be projected from it. The distance *W* between the flat sides of the hexagon should be equal to 1.5*D* + 3 mm.

Methods of preventing rotation of a bolt while screwing a nut on or off it:

When it is not possible to hold a bolt-head by means of a spanner, the bolt is prevented from rotating by the provision of one of the following, below the bolt-head:

(*i*) A square neck

(*ii*) A pin

(*iii*) A snug.

These are shown and described below while dealing with various forms of bolts.

Square-headed bolt: This bolt is generally used when the head is to be accommodated in a recess. This recess also is made of square shape so that the bolt is prevented from turning when the nut is screwed on or off it. This bolt is commonly used in bearings for shafts. The bolt-head is chamfered at its upper end.

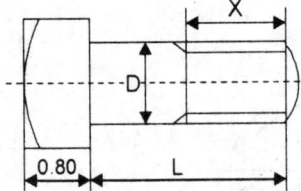 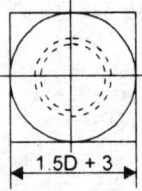

Fig. 7.5: *Square-headed bolt*

Thickness of bolt-head = 0.8*D* to *D*

Width across flats = 1.5*D* + 3 mm.

□□□

8

Rivets and Riveted Joints

The devices used for holding together the two parts of a machine or a structure are called 'Fasteners'. These fasteners vary in kind and use, from ordinary nails and glue to screwed pieces, rivets, keys and cotters, etc. varying in size for use in locomotives to watches.

CLASSIFICATION OF FASTENERS

Fasteners are divided into two main categories:

    1. Temporary fasteners   2. Permanent or semipermanent fasteners.

    Temporary fasteners allow easy unfastening of the parts connected, while with semipermanent fasteners the parts, when joined once, cannot be separated without breaking the joining element. Temporary fasteners are widely used in joining the machine parts and other engineering products where frequent dismantling is required. Nuts and bolts, screws, studs, keys, cotters and pins, etc. are examples of temporary fasteners; whereas riveting, welding, soldering and brazing, etc. are permanent fastenings.

RIVETS

Rivets are short cylindrical pieces of ductile metal with a head, formed during manufacture, at one end and a tail on the other end (Fig. 8.1). A head is formed on the other side also after the rivet has been put in place through the aligned rivet holes in the two plates to be joined. They are usually employed to fasten together pieces of sheet metal or fasten plates to rolled sections or rolled sections to each other. Rivets are made from various metals and alloys including copper, brass, aluminium, etc. Rivet is designated by giving the type of head, shank diameter and length, e.g. a snap head Rivet of 10 mm and 50 mm long is designated as Snap Head Rivet 10 × 50 (Fig. 8.1).

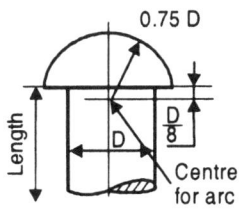

Fig. 8.1: *Easy drawing proportions for snap head rivets*

RIVETED JOINTS

These come under semipermanent type of fasteners as the joint cannot be undone without chipping off the rivet heads. Riveted joints are used in structural and machine work exposed to vibrational loads and for connecting metal elements having poor weldability, e.g. in the building of pressure vessels like boilers, hydraulic tanks, penstocks, air receivers, etc., and structures like roof-trusses, bridges and towers, etc. In general they are used when subjected to shear stresses and not to tension.

The length of rivet required to form a head varies according to the head shape. For snap and conical heads about 1.5 D is sufficient. The diameter (D) is determined from the thickness of the plates to be connected. If 't' is the thickness of the plates then by Prof. Unwin's formula $D = 6\sqrt{t}$ where 't' is in mm or $D = 1.9\sqrt{t}$ where 't' is in cm. This empirical rule is applicable only when plates and rivets are of substantial size. t may be tabulated as given in Table 8.1.

Table 8.1

Thickness of plate, t mm	8	9	10	11	12	14	16	18	20	22
Diameter of finished rivet, D mm	17	18	19	20	21	22	24	25	27	28

RIVETED JOINTS

There are two main types of riveted joints.

    1. Lap joint   2. Butt joint.

When the plates to be connected overlap each other, the joint is known as a lap joint. If the edges of the plates to be connected but against each other, the joint is known as a butt joint.

Lap joint: A single riveted lap joint is shown in pictorial view in Fig. 8.2. A lap joint is called single riveted lap joint if there is only one row of rivets passing through the two plates connected together. Similarly, it is called double riveted if there are two rows of rivets. Treble riveted if there are three rows and so on. In case of joints having two or more rows. The rivets in adjoining rows can be arranged in chain formation, i.e. opposite each other, or in zigzag staggered formation.

Diameter of the rivet (d) = 6 $\sqrt{t}$

Where t = thickness of the plates to be connected in mm.

The value of the diameter so obtained is rounded to the nearest standard size of rivets. The standard sizes in for rivet diameters recommended by the Indian standard are as follows:

        12, 14, 16, 18, 20, 22, 24, 27, 30, 33, 36, 39, 42, 48.

Pitch(p) = 3d

Where p = distance between the axes of adjoining rivets in the same row measured parallel to the edges of the plates.

Distance between an edge of the plate and the nearest rivet axis = $1.5d$. The distance between the edge of the plate and the nearest rivet hole is obviously equal to diameter d. This distance is known as the margin m.

Single-riveted lap joint: Sectional elevation and plan of a single-riveted lap joint drawn using the above rules is shown in the figure represents only a part of large plates and hence, three edges of each plate are shown by break lines.

Double-riveted lap joint: Double-riveted joints may be of chain type, or zigzag type. In case of chain type, the rivets in adjoining rows are opposite to each other. In zigzag, the rivets in adjoining rows are staggered.

The distance between two rows is known as row pitch (p_r). The minimum value of p_r is $2d$ in zigzag type and $2d + 6$ mm in chain types.

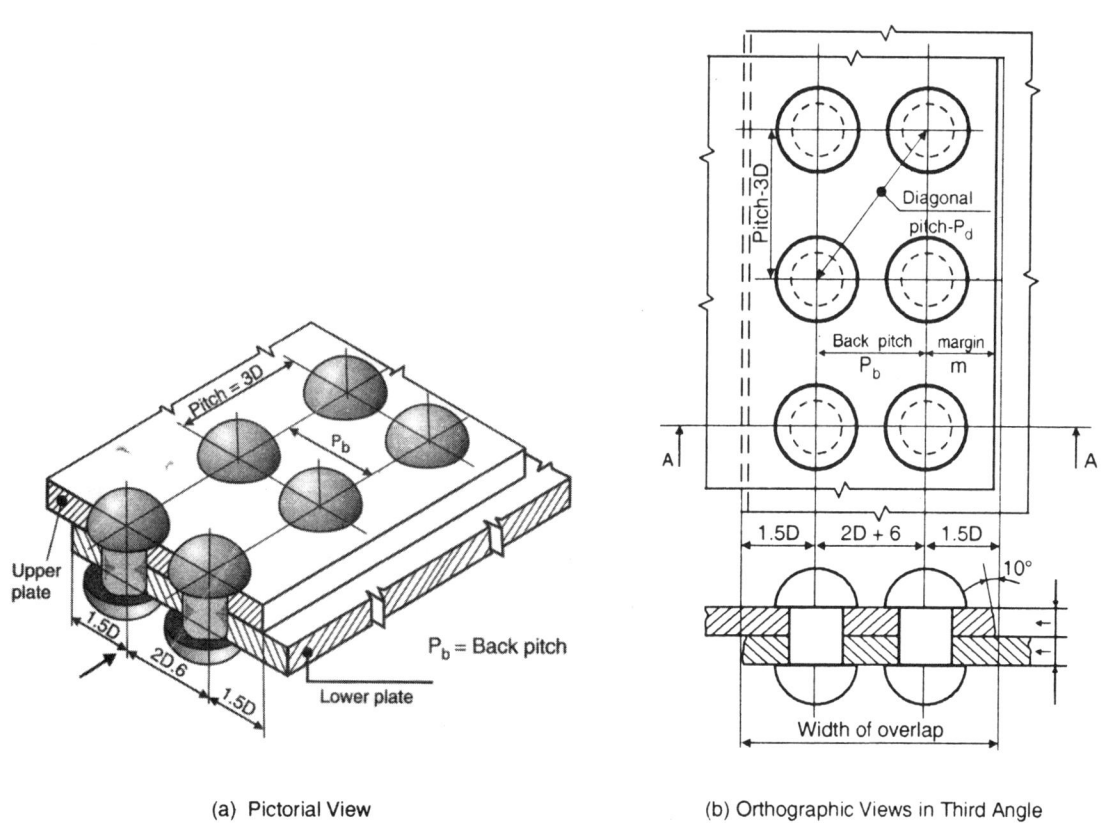

| (a) Pictorial View | (b) Orthographic Views in Third Angle |

Fig. 8.2: *Double riveted lap joint (chain riveting)*

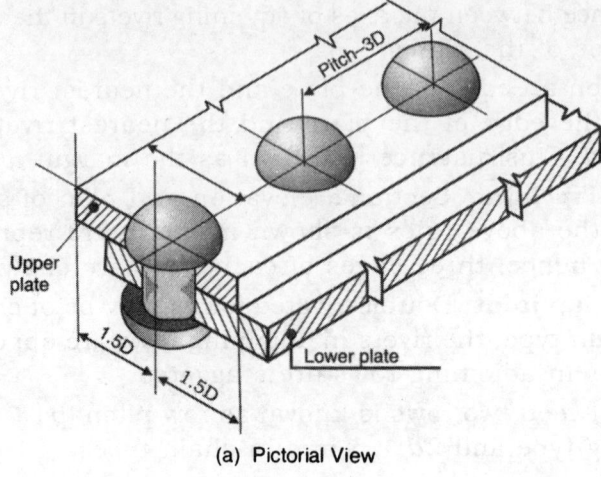

(a) Pictorial View

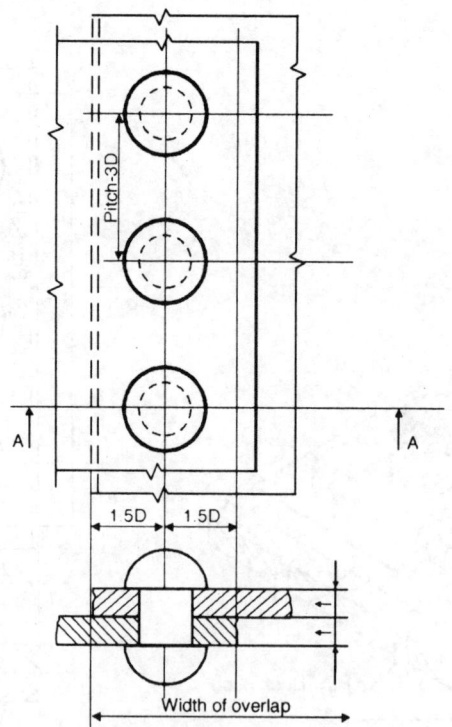

(b) Orthographic Views in Third Angle

Fig. 8.3 : *Single riveted lap joint (chain riveting)*

□ □ □

9

Sectioned Views

Sometimes the full details of the object cannot be obtained by outside views only. In such situations, the object is imagined to be cut by a plane, called *section plane* or *cutting plane* (CP) and the cut-away part is discarded and the view (plan, elevation, or side view) of the remaining part is drawn. This way interior detail can be easily shown. The portion over which the imaginary cutting plane has passed is shown by thin lines drawn at some angle (usually 45°) to the main outlines. These lines are called *section lines* or *hatching lines*. These lines must be drawn by 2H pencil. The cutting plane is indicated by cutting plane line (thick tong dash and two short dashes) and is designated by capital letters and the direction of viewing is shown by two arrows resting on it. It must always be remembered that the cutting plane is imaginary, and it doesn't affect other views.

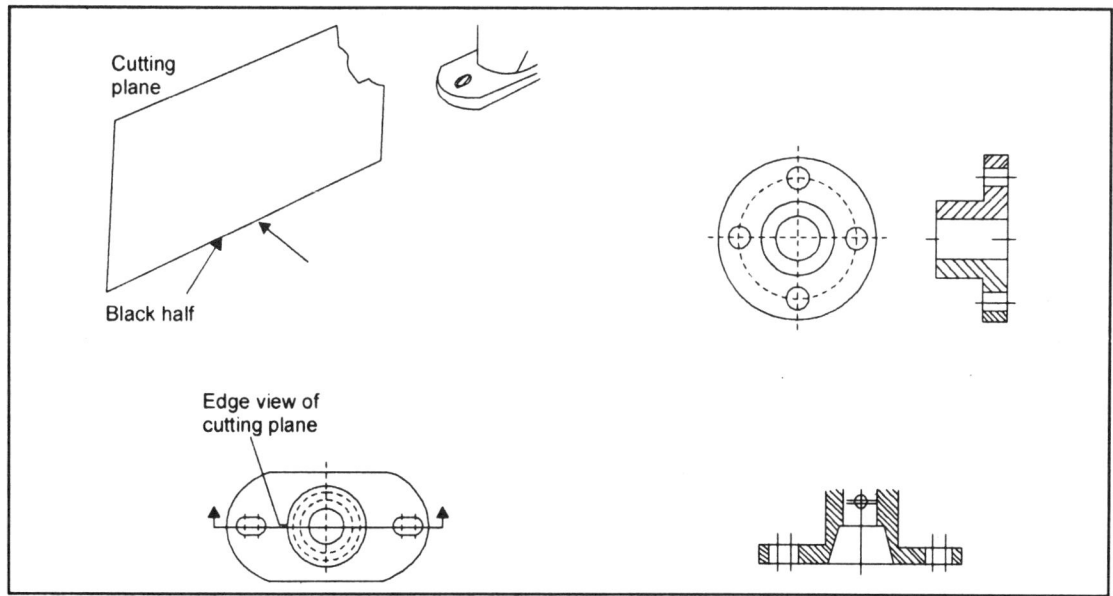

Fig. 9.1

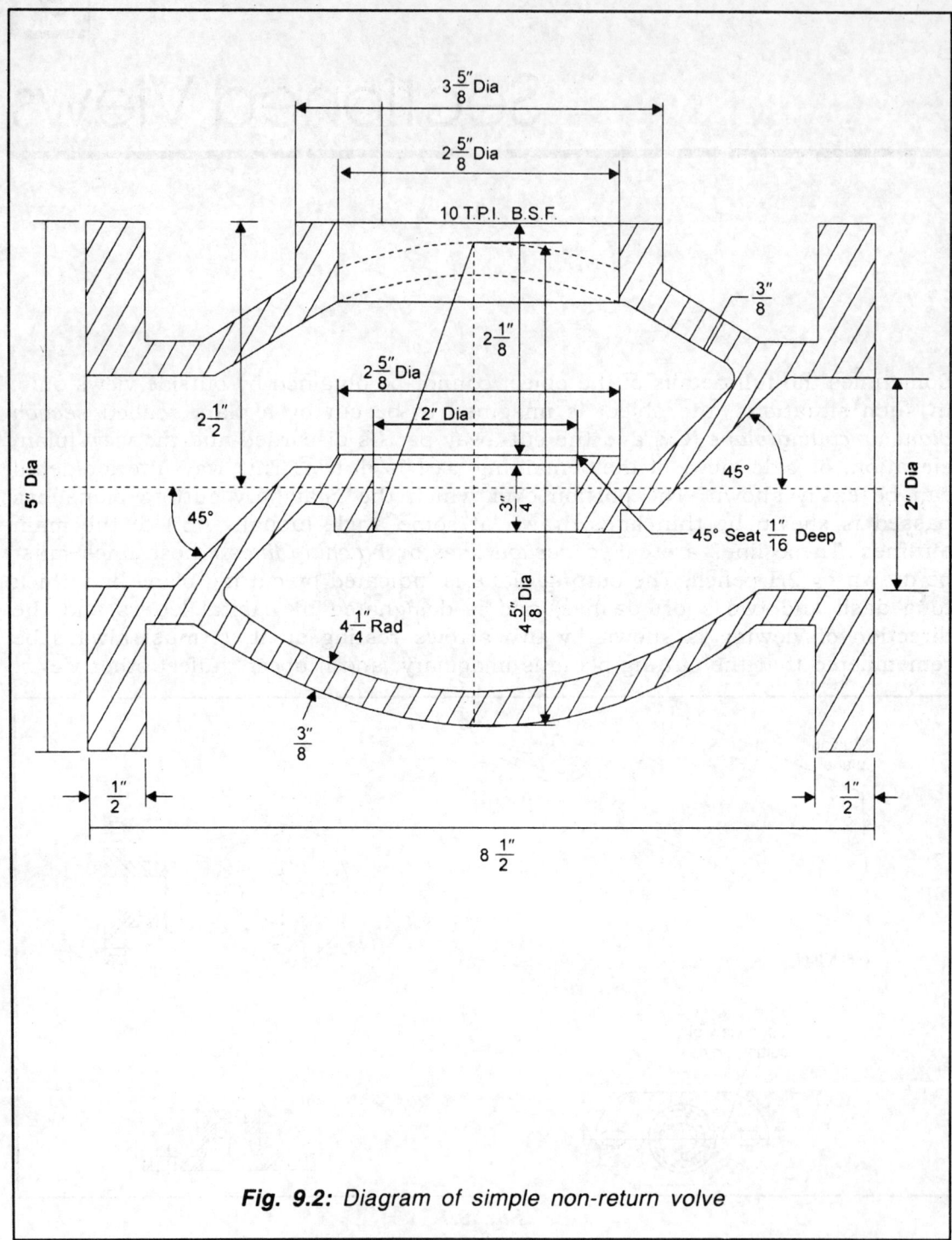

Fig. 9.2: *Diagram of simple non-return volve*

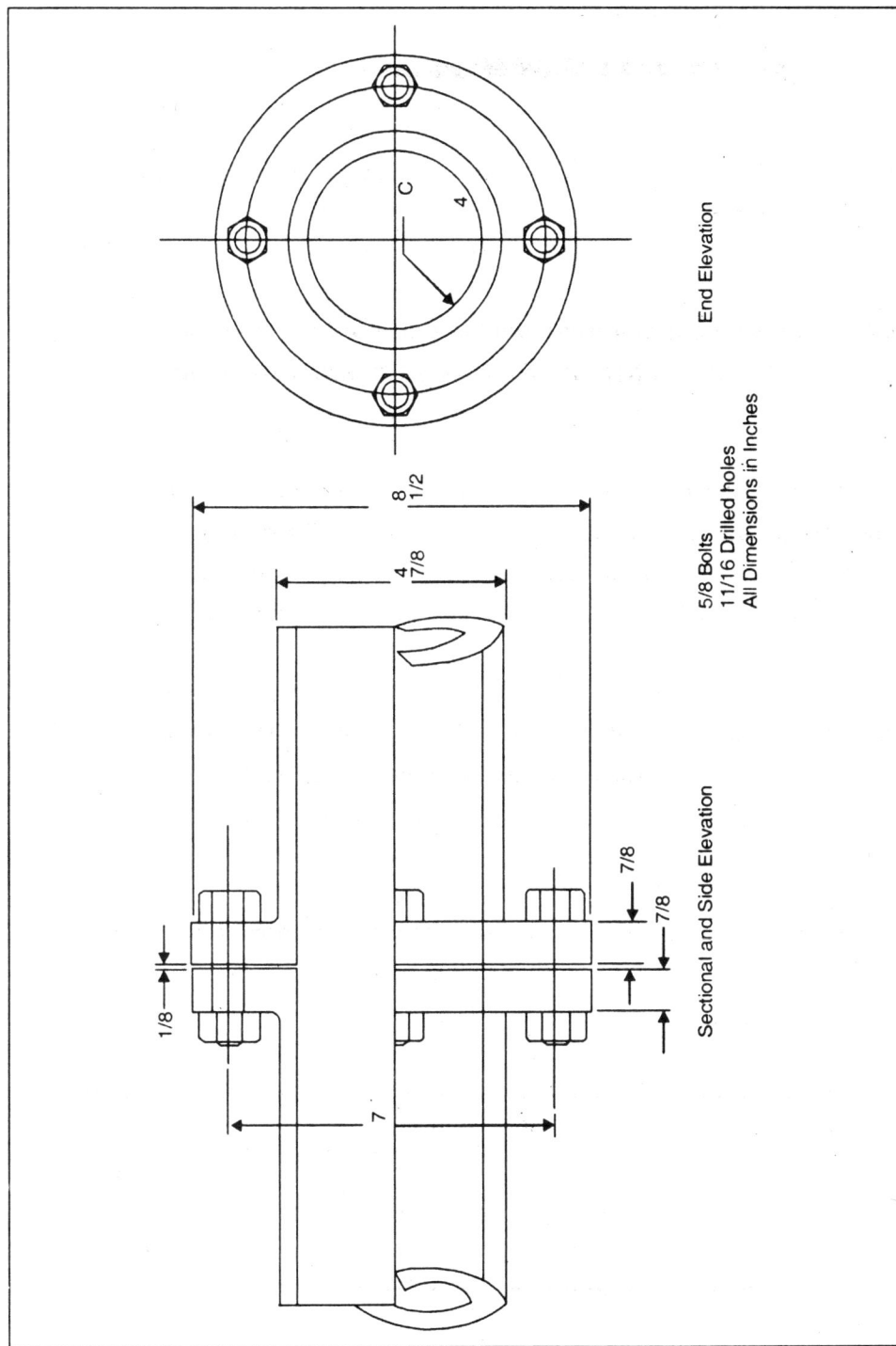

End Elevation

Sectional and Side Elevation

5/8 Bolts
11/16 Drilled holes
All Dimensions in Inches

Fig. 9.3: Cast iron pipes and joint

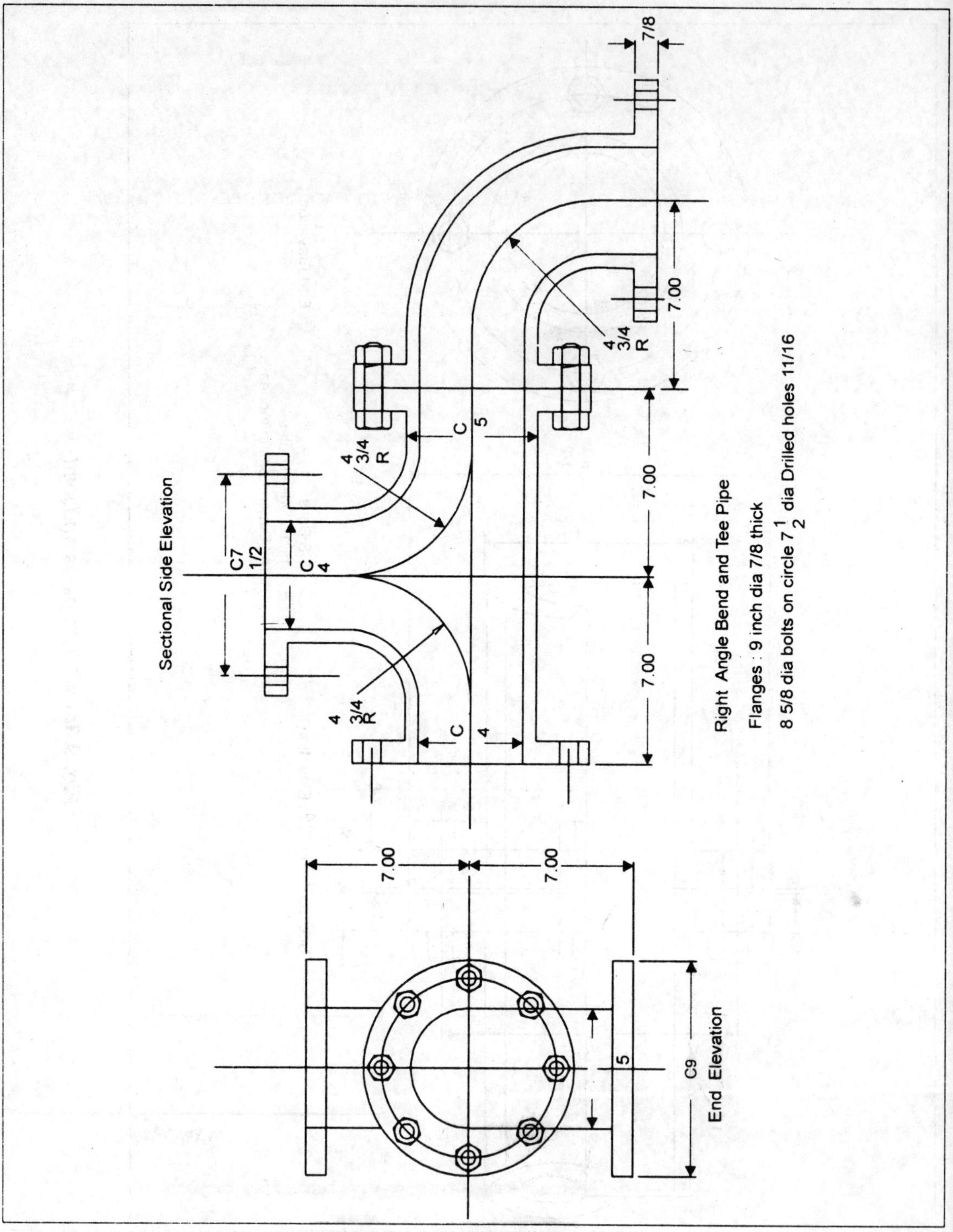

Sectional Side Elevation

C7 1/2
C 4
3/4 R
3/4 R
C
4
5
C

7.00
7.00
7.00
7/8
4 3/4 R

End Elevation

7.00
7.00
5
C9

Right Angle Bend and Tee Pipe

Flanges : 9 inch dia 7/8 thick

8 5/8 dia bolts on circle $7\frac{1}{2}$ dia Drilled holes 11/16

10

Blue Prints,
Flow Diagrams and Machines

Engineering drawings are also referred as blueprints/bluelines. Most copies of engineering drawings that were formerly made by using a chemical printing process that yielded graphics on blue-coloured paper or blue lines on white paper with the help of ammonia. Therefore they are also known as ammonia prints. Now-a-days, the mechanics of the drafting task have largely been automated and accelerated through the use of Computer Aided Design System (CAD) which has served to enlarge the skill set required by today's designer and drafters.

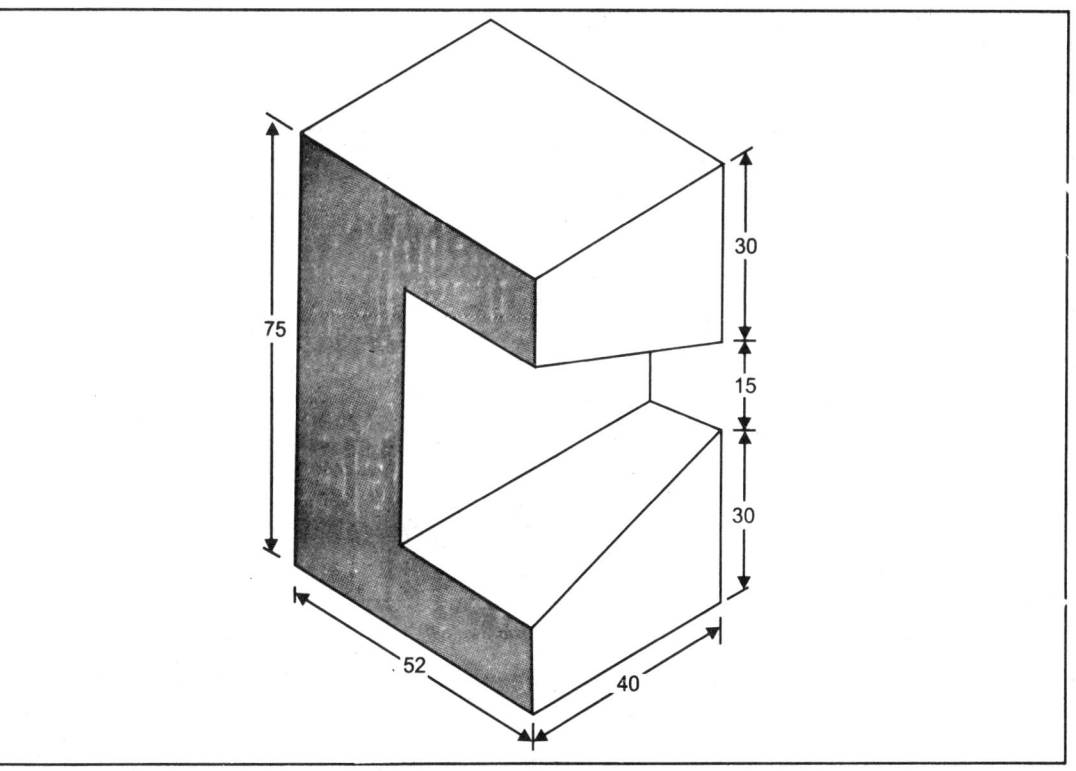

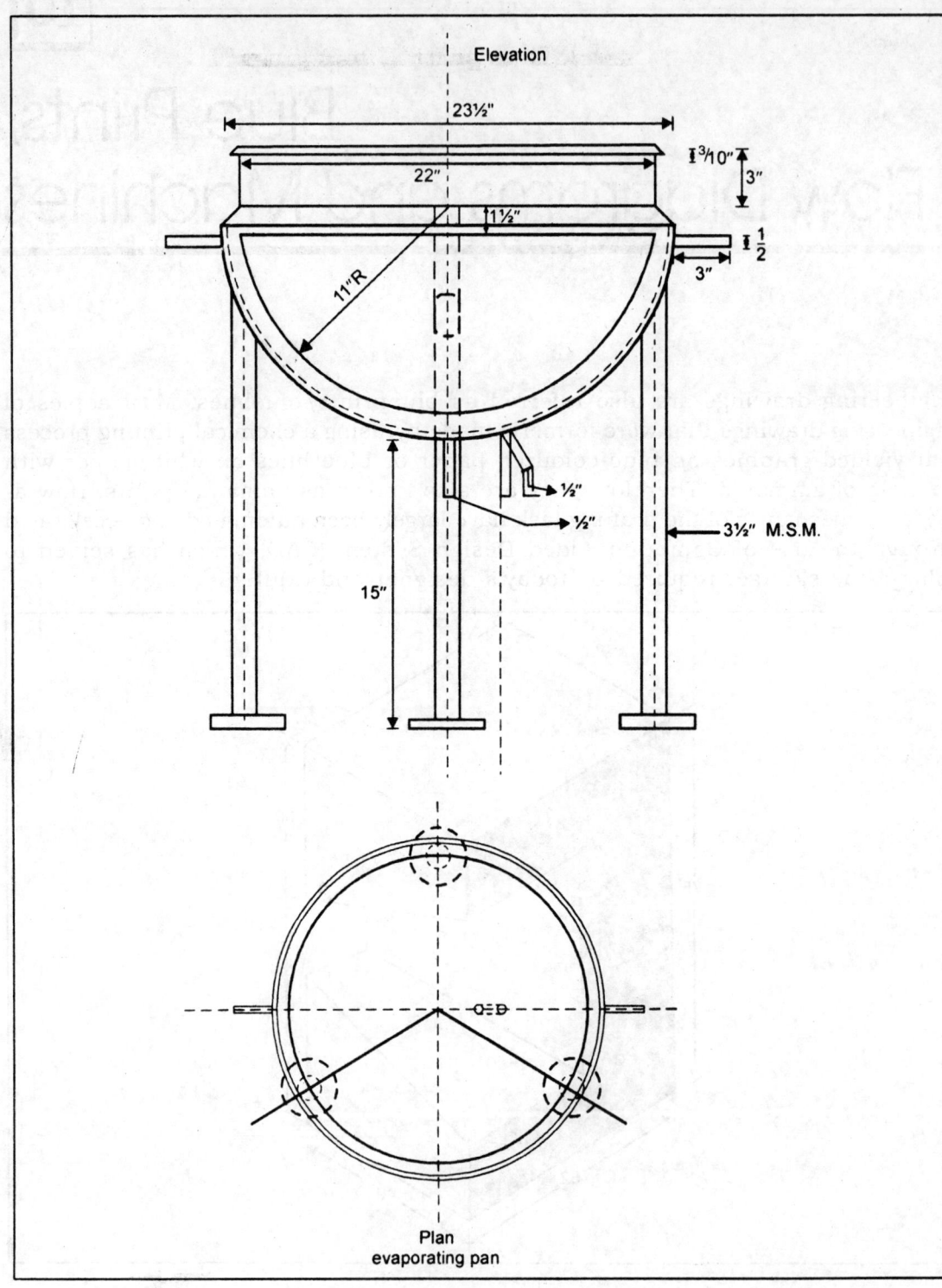

Elevation

23½"

22"

1³⁄₁₀"

3"

1½"

11"R

½"

½"

½

3"

3½" M.S.M.

15"

Plan
evaporating pan

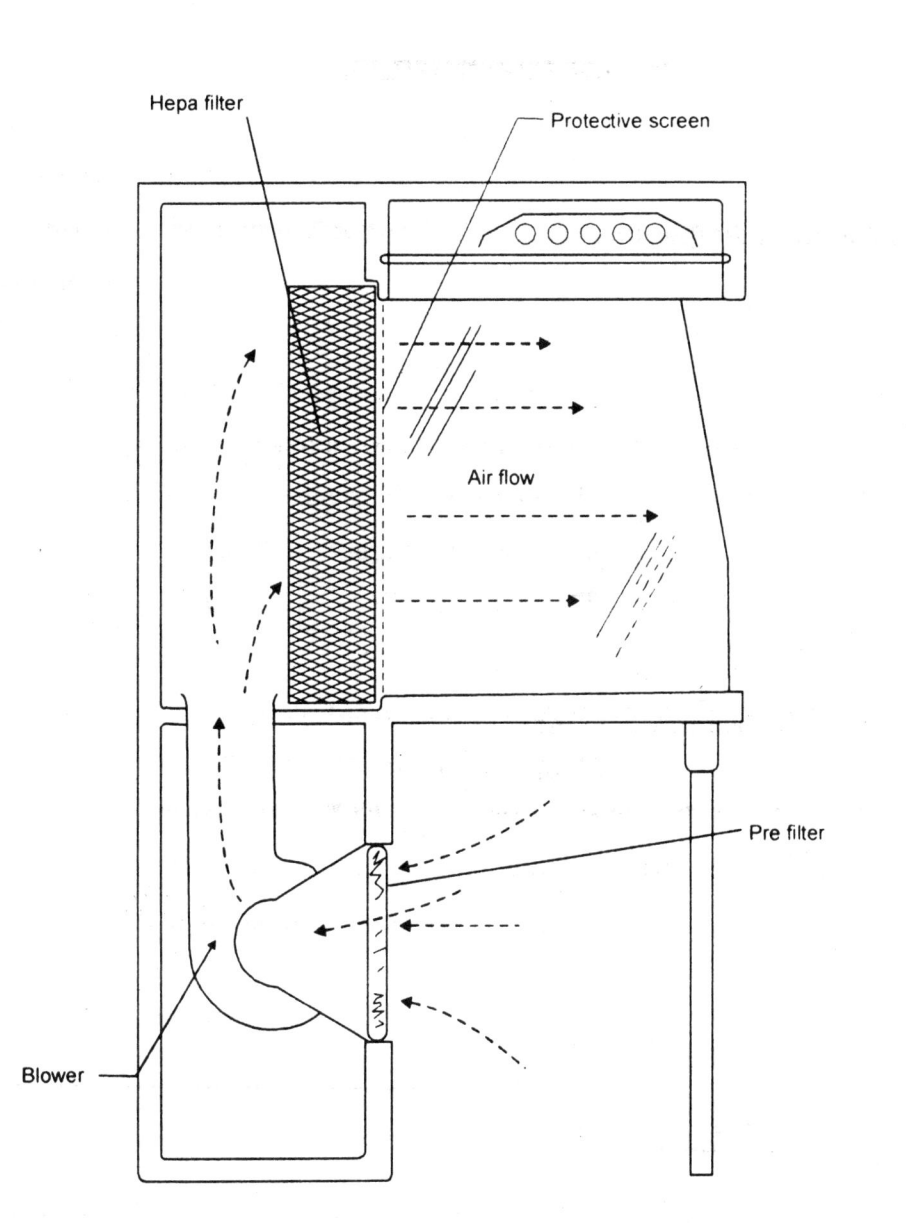

Hepa filter

Protective screen

Air flow

Pre filter

Blower

Horizontal laminar-flow workbench

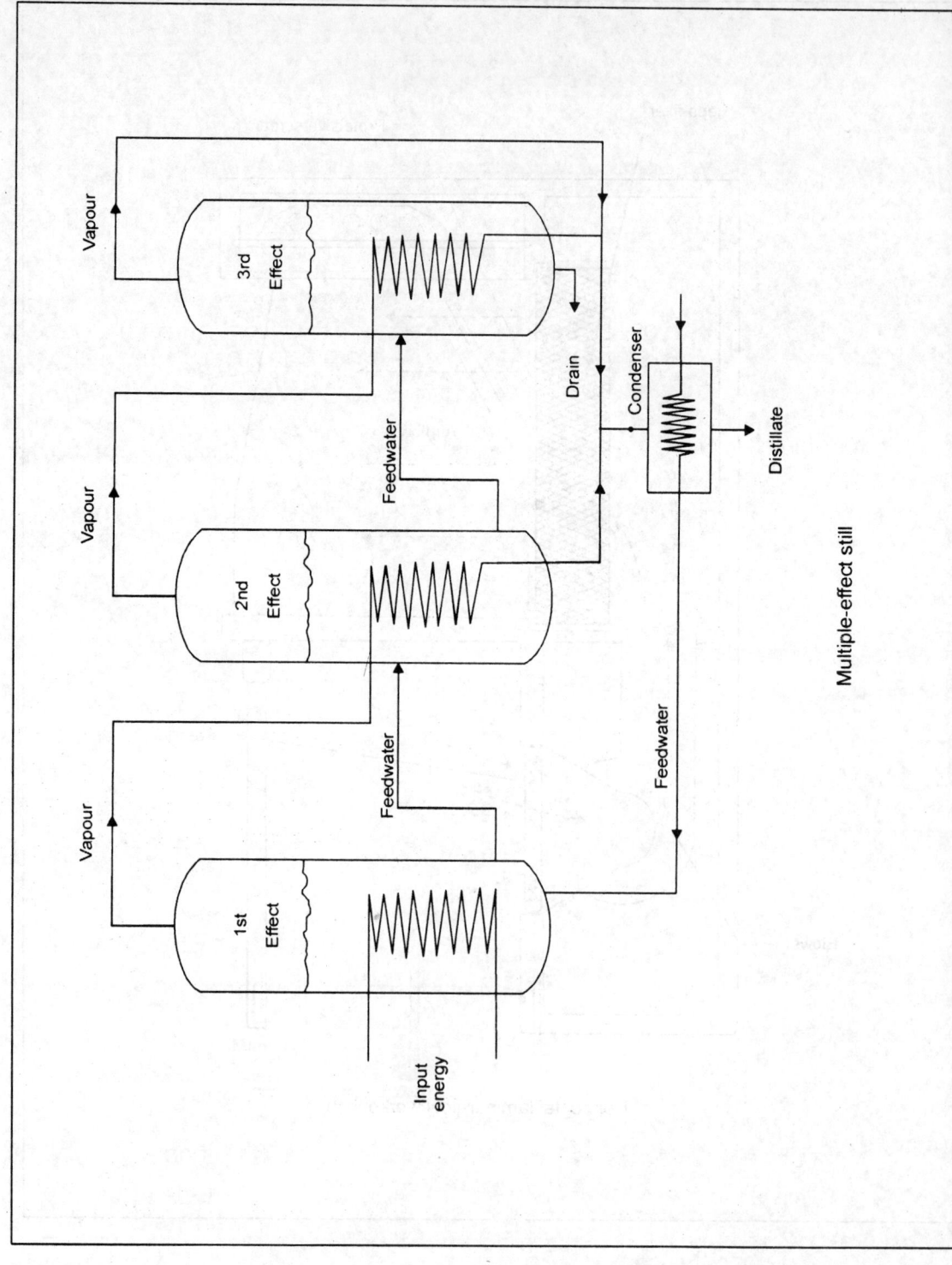

Multiple-effect still

FLOW CHART

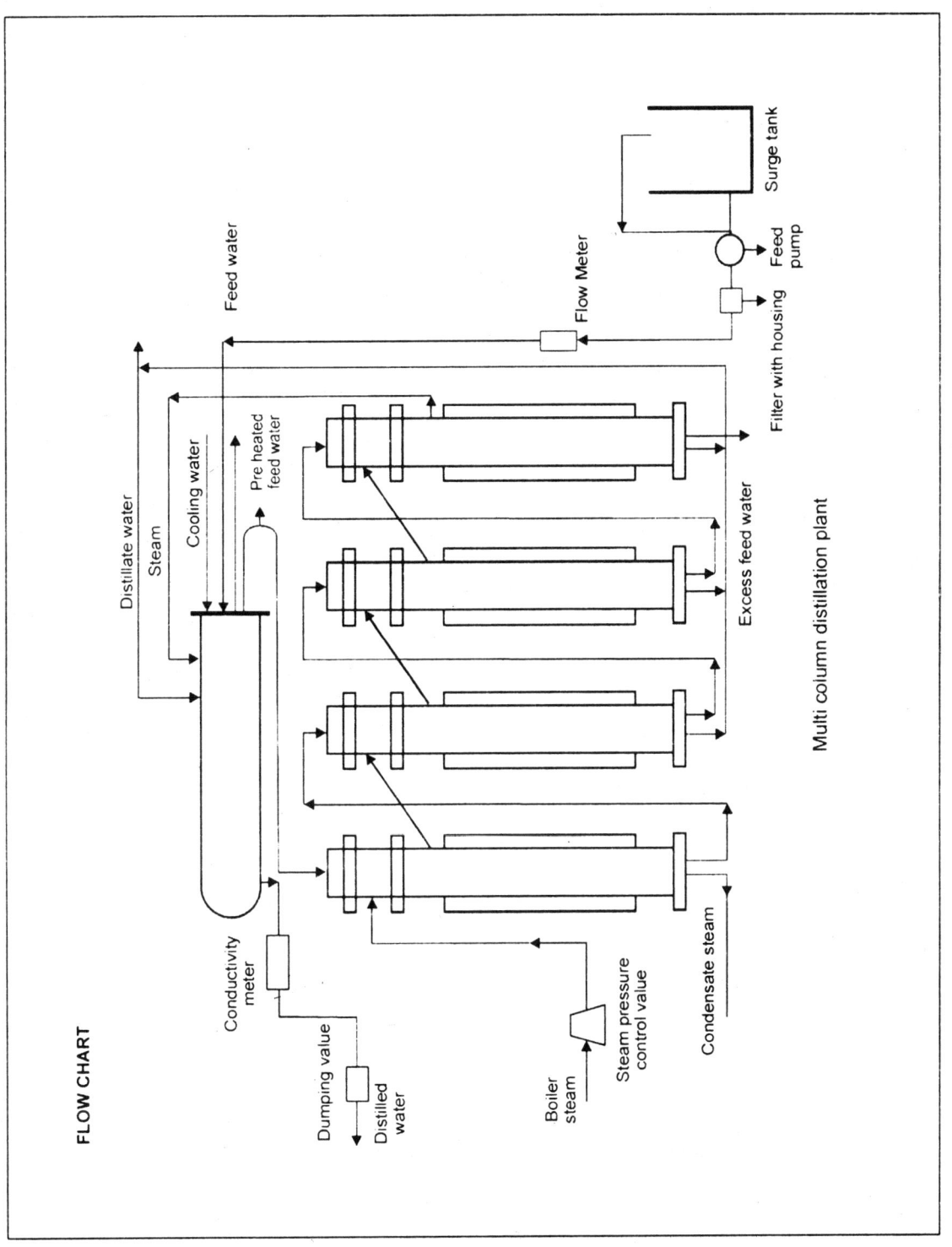

Multi column distillation plant

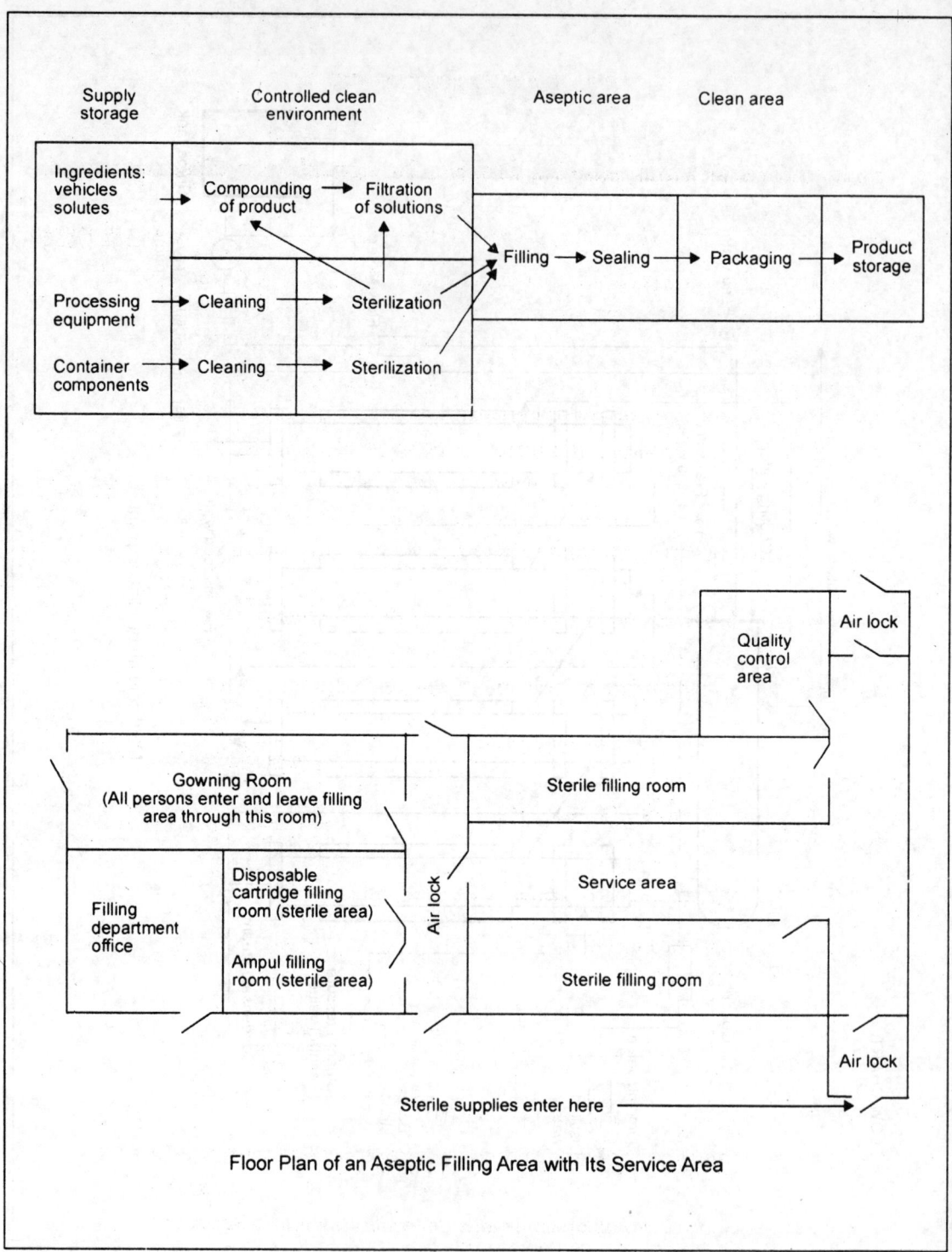

Floor Plan of an Aseptic Filling Area with Its Service Area

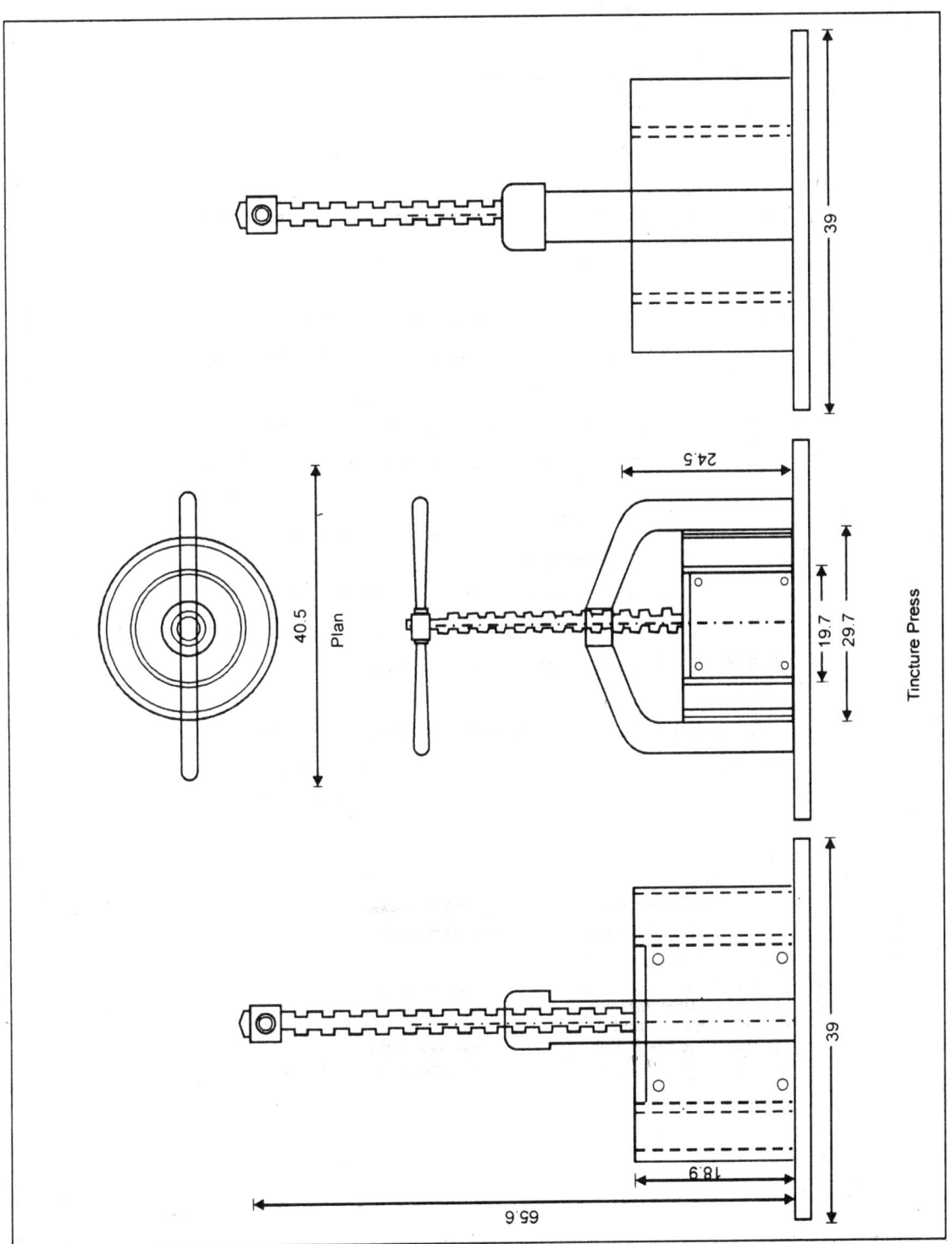

Tincture Press

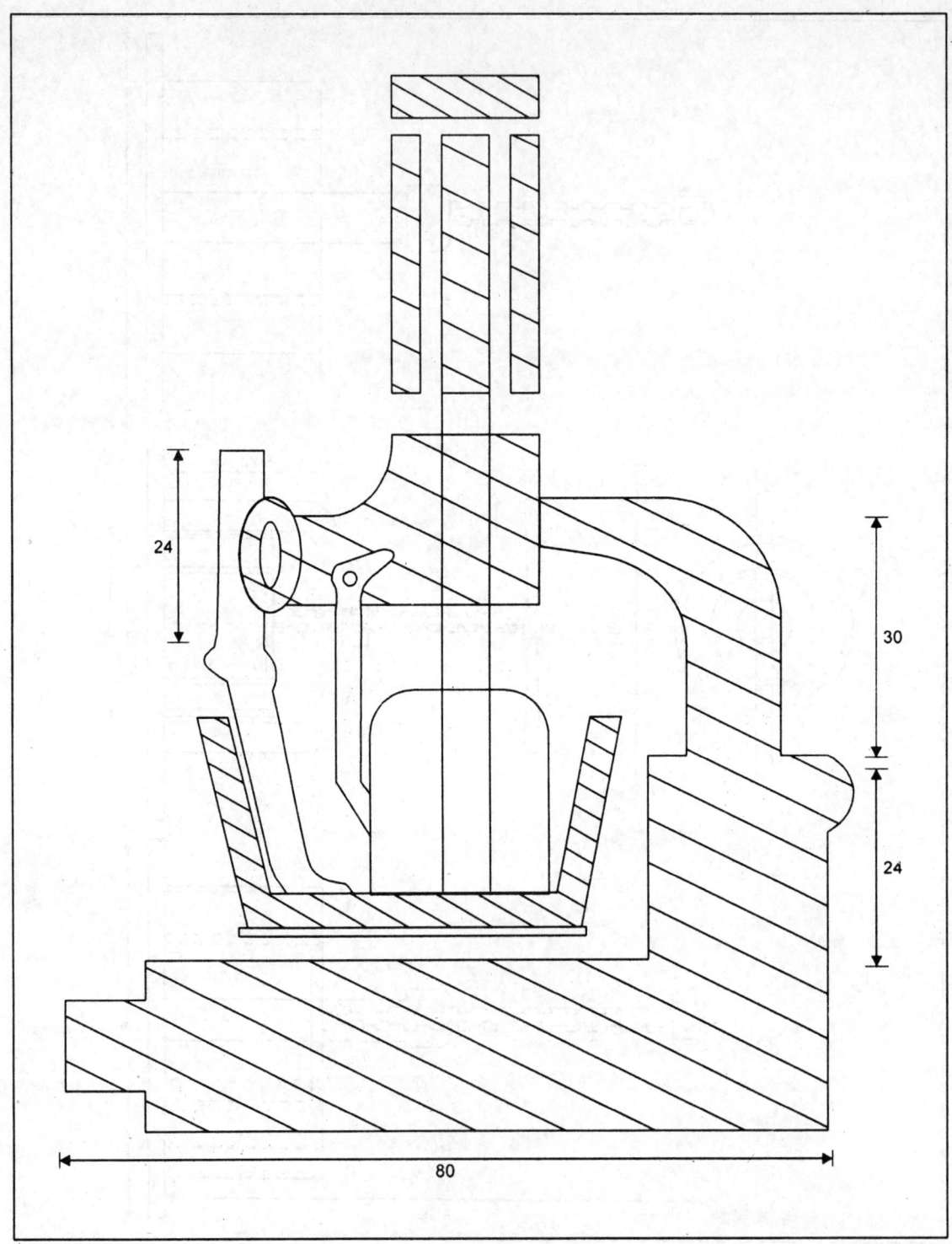

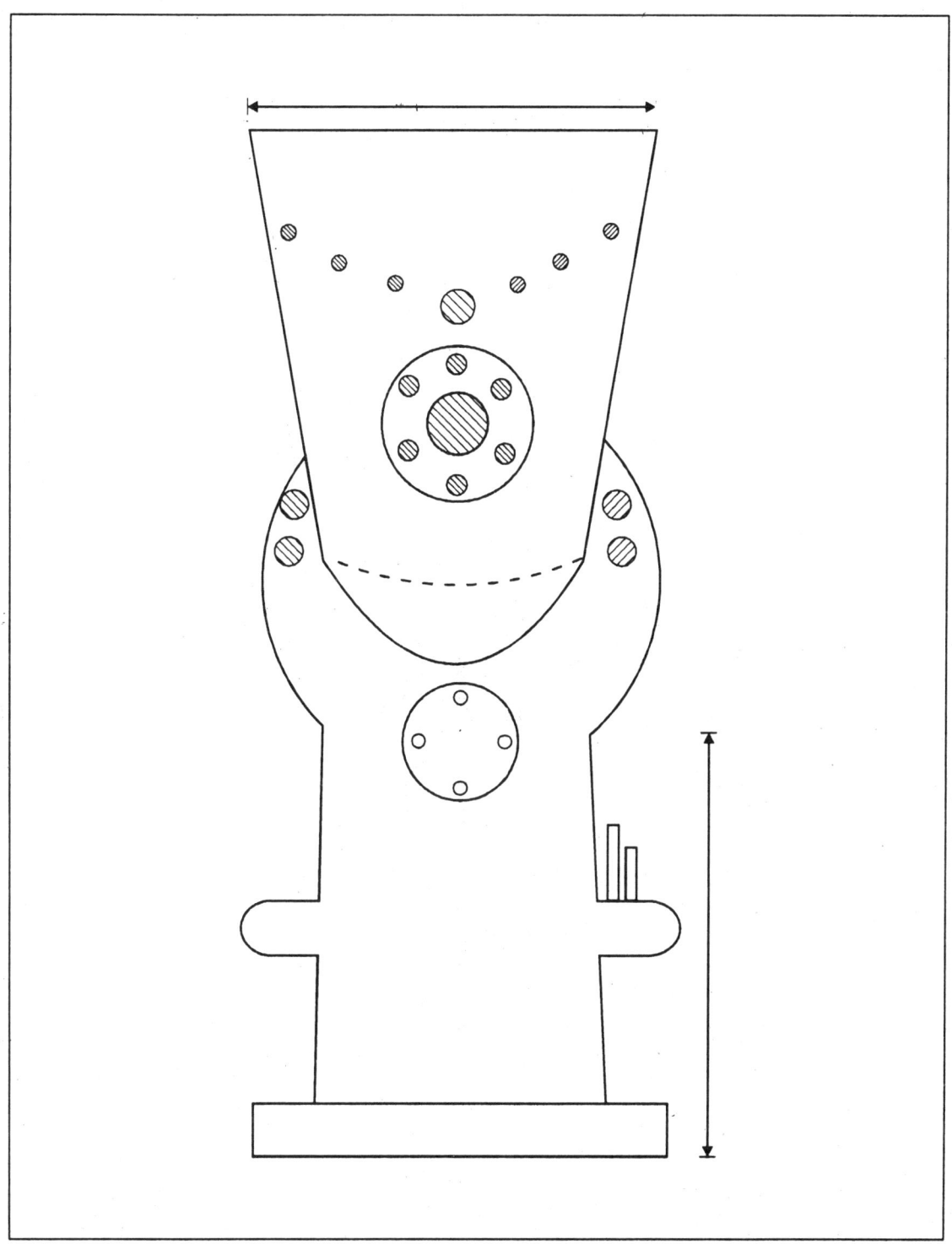

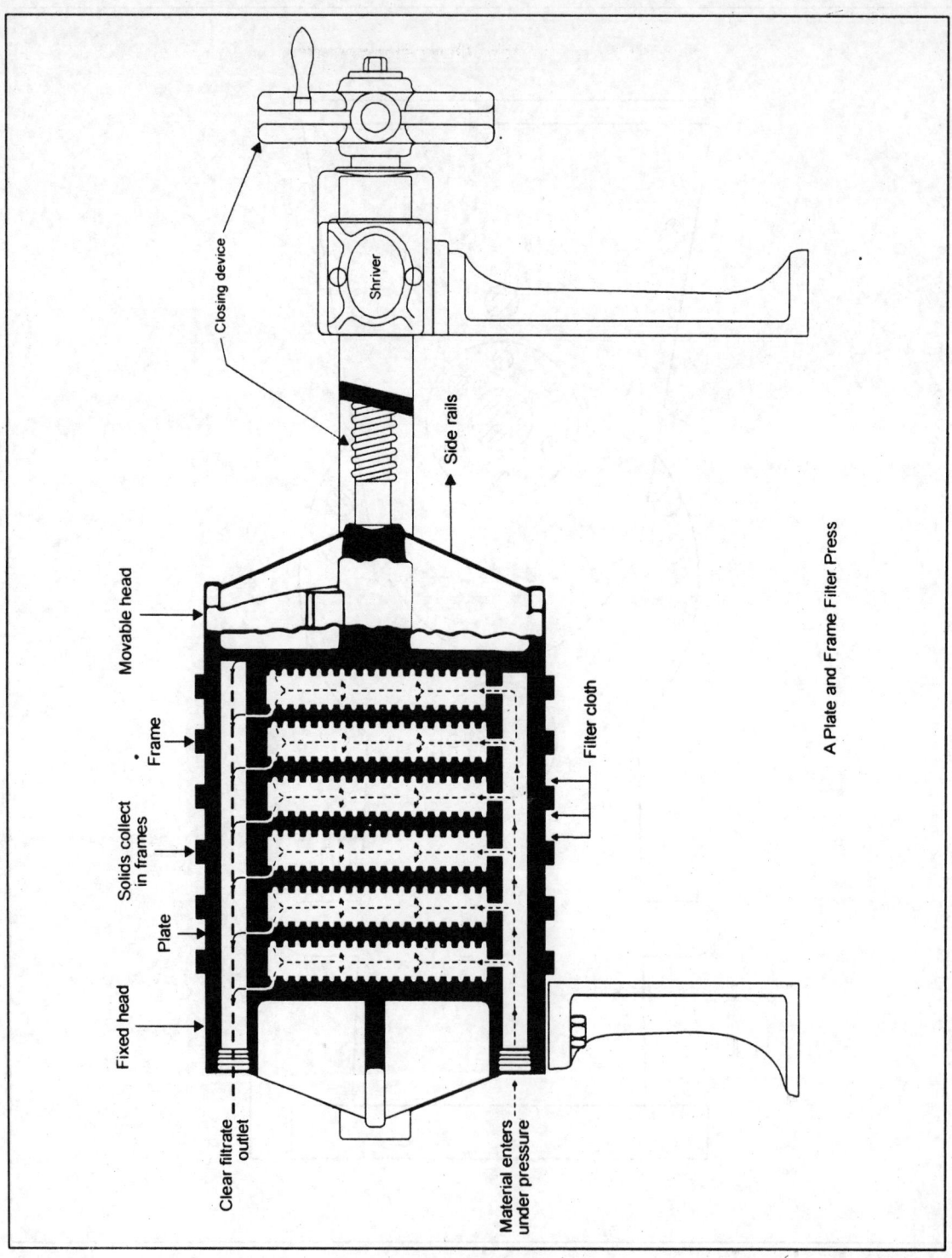

Closing device

Shriver

Side rails

Movable head

Frame

Solids collect
in frames

Plate

Fixed head

Filter cloth

Clear filtrate
outlet

Material enters
under pressure

A Plate and Frame Filter Press

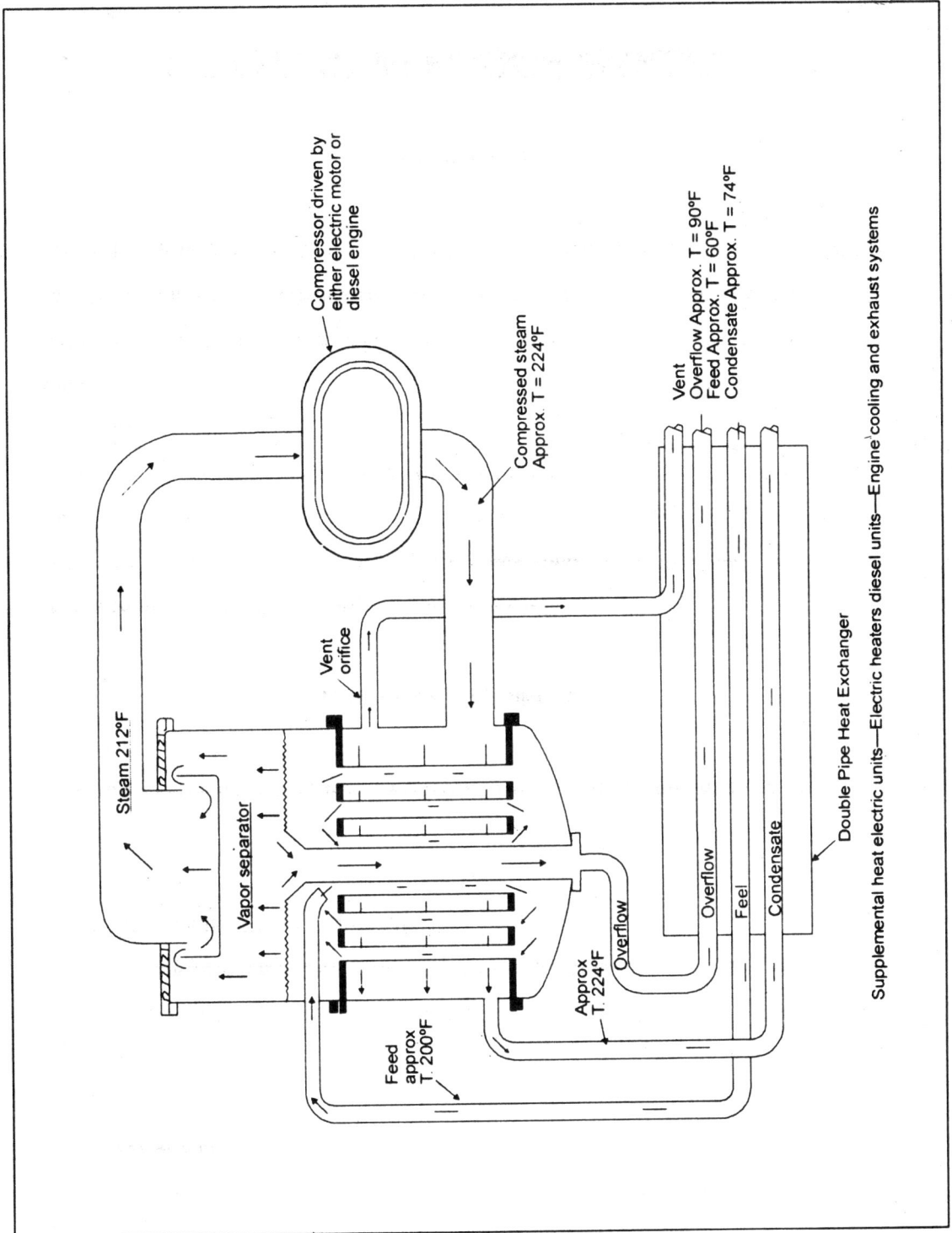

Compressor driven by either electric motor or diesel engine

Compressed steam Approx. T = 224°F

Vent
Overflow Approx. T = 90°F
Feed Approx. T = 60°F
Condensate Approx. T = 74°F

Vent orifice

Steam 212°F

Vapor separator

Overflow

Feel

Condensate

Double Pipe Heat Exchanger

Feed approx T. 200°F

Approx T. 224°F

Overflow

Supplemental heat electric units—Electric heaters diesel units—Engine cooling and exhaust systems

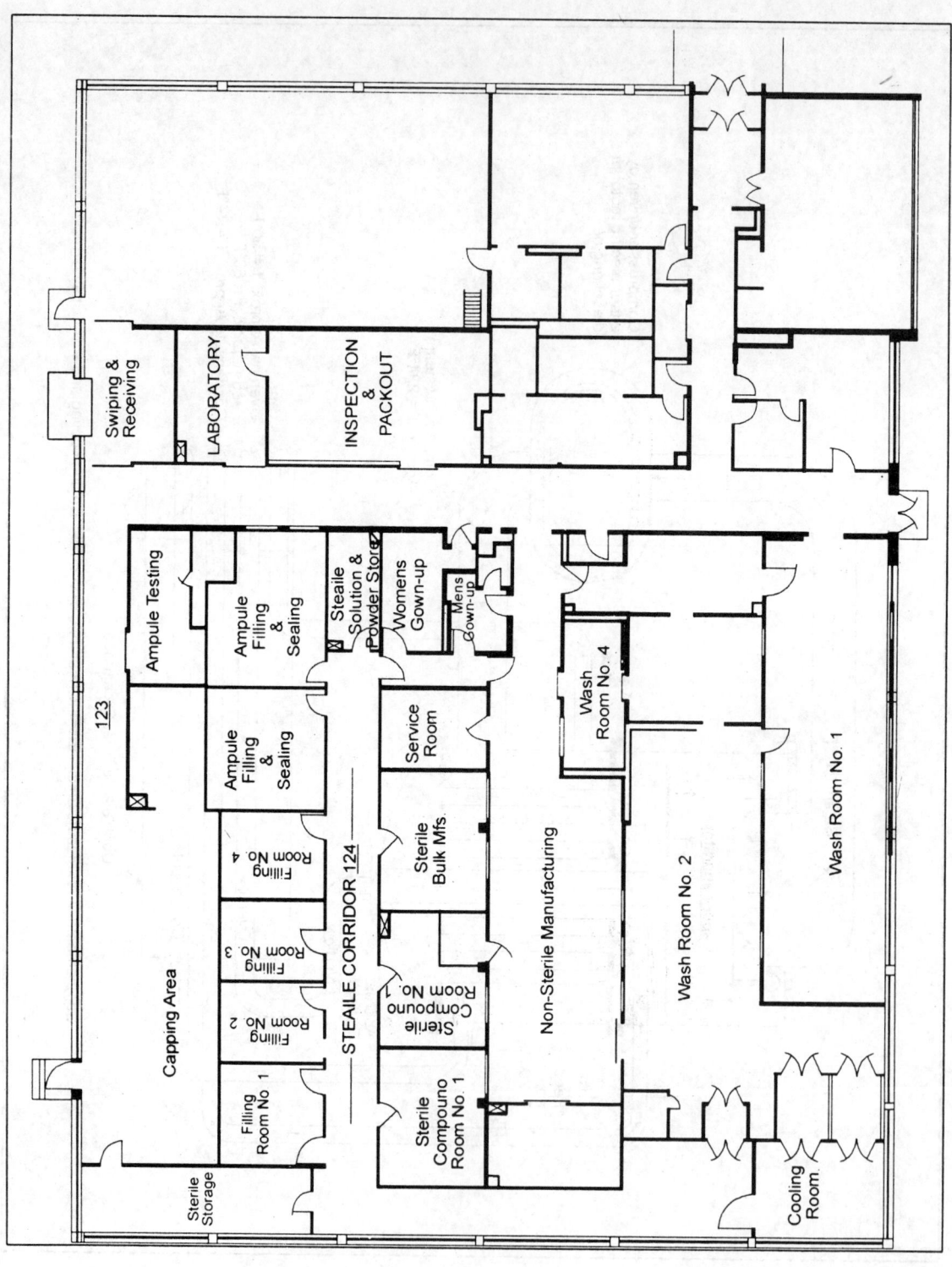

11

Units of Measurement and their Conversion

1 centimetre (cm)	= 10 millimetre (mm)	= 0.3937 inch
1 decametre (dm)	= 10 centimetre	= 3.94 inch
1 metre (m)	= 10 decametre	= 100 centimetre
1 kilometre (km)	= 1000 metre	= 0.6214 mile
1 inch (in.)	= 2.54 centimetre	= 25.4 millimetre
1 foot (ft)	= 12 inch	= 0.3048 metre
1 yard (yd)	= 3 feet	= 0.9144 metre
1 rod (rd)	= 5.5 yards	
1 mile (mi)	= 1760 yards	= 1.609 kilometre
1 square cm	= 100 sq mm (mm^2)	
1 sq m (m^2)	= 10,000 sq cm (cm^2)	
1 hectare	= 10,000 sq m (m^2)	
1 sq km	= 1,000,000 sq m (m^2)	
1 sq foot(ft^2)	= 144 sq inch (in^2)	
1 sq yard (yd^2)	= 9 sq feet (ft^2)	
1 acre	= 4,840 sq yards (yd^2)	
1 sq mile (mi^2)	= 640 acres	

To convert	into	multiply by
cm	in	0.3937
m	feet	3.281
km	mile	0.6214
m	yard	1.0940
inch	cm	2.5400
feet	m	0.3048
mile	km	1.6050
yards	m	0.9144
sq inches	sq cm	6.4520
sq feet	sq m	0.0929
acres	hectares	0.4047
sq miles	sq km	2.5900
sq yards	sq m	0.8361
sq inches	sq cm	6.4520
sq feets	sq m	0.0929